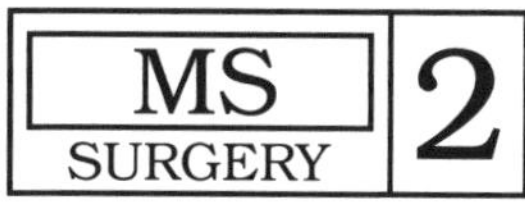

Master Series in Surgery

Series Editor:
Dana K. Andersen, MD

Advance *noun*....progress, improvement, movement toward a goal.

Each volume in the Master Series in Surgery *will provide a comprehensive review of current advances in a major area of surgery. The objective is to provide the reader with practical, up-to-date information and to favor the clinical more than the experimental aspect of the topics presented. However, special attention will be devoted to the discussion of recent investigative findings that might impact the conduct of surgical and clinical practices in these areas. The volumes of the series are not intended to serve as "how-to" books, but as useful references by authorities in the field.*

Series Editor: Dana K. Andersen, MD

Forthcoming Volumes:

Volume 3 Advances in Colorectal Carcinoma Surgery
Volume 4 Advances in Wound Healing and Tissue Repair

Advances in Surgery in the Elderly

Volume 2

Master Series in Surgery

Series Editor: Dana K. Andersen, MD
Professor of Surgery and Medicine
Chief, Section of General Surgery
Department of Surgery
The University of Chicago

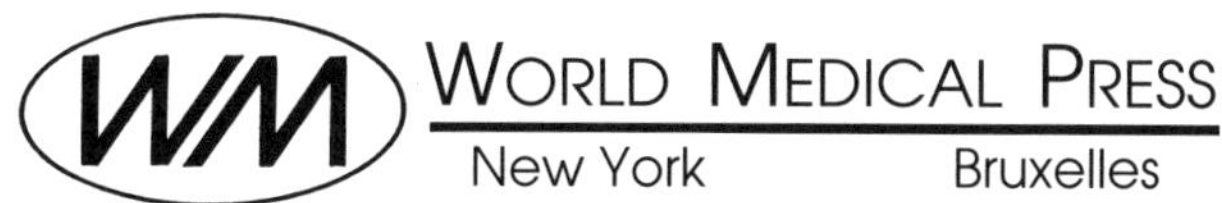

Library of Congress Cataloging in Publication Data
Main entry under title:
Advances in Surgery in the Elderly
(Master Series in Surgery)
Include bibliographies and index.

Printed in the United States of America

ISBN 0-933751-03-6 World Medical Press New York/Bruxelles

Preface

TO VOLUME 2

In the early years of this century "elderly" surgical patients were defined as those over the age of 50 years. Today, reports of surgery in patients over the age of 90 or even 100 years are viewed with little surprise. During the past two decades geriatric surgical disease has increased more than any other category of activity, and has been principally responsible for the increased workload of the average general surgeon. With the transition of the post–World War II "baby boomers" from middle aged to elderly status, this trend will only increase.

Thus, geriatric surgery has emerged as a special interest that is no longer limited to broken hips and bedsores. The pathophysiology of some surgical conditions is unique in elderly patients, and the management of common surgical problems is frequently complex due to coexisting disease. The successful management of elderly patients requires considerable knowledge, careful judgment, and the avoidance of assumptions.

Age, per se, is no longer a contraindication to surgical treatment. Improved surgical results in the elderly have come about from better perioperative care, based upon an understanding of the pathophysiology of normal aging. An awareness of age-related changes in various organ systems, and an increased ability to monitor these systems, also has contributed to improved outcomes. In addition, our awareness of coexisting diseases or impairments, and our ability to effectively compensate for these limitations has resulted in surgical outcomes in some elderly patients that are virtually the same as those in younger patients.

Perhaps the most important statistic a surgeon can have at his or her fingertips is the life expectancy for a patient of any given age. In the section on general considerations we learn that a 70-year-old patient has an average life expectancy of 13 years. Therefore, a correctable, potentially life-threatening illness should be addressed in such a patient if the risk of operation is acceptable. The next most important statistic for a surgeon is the relationship of the risk of emergency surgery to that of elective surgery. For most conditions, emergency surgery carries a perioperative mortality risk at least threefold greater than that of elective surgery. Conditions that are treated easily in the elective setting can degenerate into potential disaster when a crisis is allowed to develop. We now appreciate that the "conservative" approach to surgical problems in elderly patients is usually an aggressive approach.

In the sections that follow, a variety of specific diseases and concerns are highlighted, and attention is drawn to unusual presentations of disease or special considerations required of the general surgeon treating an elderly patient. In the section on gastrointestinal disease, the etiology and treatment of esophageal, gastroduodenal, and intestinal conditions are reviewed. The atypical and high-risk presentation of duodenal and gastric ulcer disease is emphasized, as is the challenge of diagnosis and treatment of small-bowel obstruction. We are reminded that one third of patients with presumed malignant obstruction actually have benign causes amenable to surgical treatment. The atypical etiology of some disorders, such as lower gastrointestinal bleeding, or the atypical signs and symptoms of disease, such as those in appendicitis, are also stressed.

The section on biliary and pancreatic disease is especially pertinent, as biliary tract disease is the single leading cause of emergency surgery in elderly patients. The pathophysiology of the dramatic increase in biliary calculus disease in the elderly is reviewed carefully. The atypical nature of the presenting signs and symptoms is stressed, as are the dire consequences of delayed treatment and nonoperative approaches to complications. On the other hand, some disease states, such as acute pancreatitis, are noteworthy for the validity of a treatment approach that is the same for younger patients as for the elderly. Common surgical problems encountered by all general surgeons are reviewed, and provide a perspective based upon recent investigation.

Our editors of the second volume of the *Master Series in Surgery* are all leading experts in their field. Their insights and discussions provide a treasure of pearls for young and experienced surgeons alike.

Michael E. Zenilman, MD, is a recognized expert in geriatric surgery and gastrointestinal physiology. In his section, Dr Zenilman reviews the demographics of our changing patient population and the implications for general surgical practice in the years ahead. Physiologic and pathophysiologic aspects of aging are reviewed, and special considerations in the preoperative care of elderly patients are discussed. The comparative outcomes of patients undergoing elective and emergency surgical treatment are discussed as well, as are the criteria by which consultation and recommendations regarding surgical disease in the elderly can be most useful.

Ronnie A. Rosenthal, MD, has published extensively in the area of surgery in the elderly, and on special considerations in the treatment of abdominal diseases in elderly patients. In her section, Dr Rosenthal reviews common disorders of the esophageal, gastroduodenal, and intestinal regions. Her discussion focuses upon conditions that are characterized by an atypical presentation or that have a particularly high likelihood of successful surgical treatment.

Joel J. Roslyn, MD, is an expert in biliary physiology and hepatobiliary surgery. In his section, Dr Roslyn reviews the pathophysiology of biliary calculus disease and explains its remarkable incidence in elderly patients. With his coauthor, **Kim U. Kahng, MD,** he analyzes approaches to treatment of common hepatobiliary and pancreatic disorders in elderly patients.

Dana K. Andersen, MD

Contributors

Series Editor:

Dana K. Andersen, MD
Professor of Surgery and Medicine
Chief, Section of General Surgery
Department of Surgery
The University of Chicago

Volume Editors:

Michael E. Zenilman, MD
Assistant Professor of Surgery
Department of Surgery
Johns Hopkins University
Francis Scott Key Medical Center

Ronnie Ann Rosenthal, MD
Associate Professor of Clinical Surgery
Department of Surgery
The University of Chicago

Joel J. Roslyn, MD
Professor and Chairman
Department of Surgery
The Medical College of Pennsylvania

Kim U. Kahng, MD
Associate Professor
Department of Surgery
The Medical College of Pennsylvania

Contents

I Considerations in Surgery in the Elderly

Michael E. Zenilman, MD

BRIEF CONTENTS

INTRODUCTION

Over the last generation the population of the United States has increased markedly, largely as a result of prolonged survival of the elderly. Intensive medical research on aging has led to improved care of elderly patients and has increased life expectancy significantly.[1] As a result, the proportion of elderly people (those over 65 years of age) in our population is increasing, and they are expected to comprise more than one quarter of the population by the year 2025.[2]

As the population ages, the survivors will approach the limit of aging, termed the life span, or maximum survival potential. Although reports exist of people living to between 120 and 130 years, the calculated life span of humans is a matter of debate,

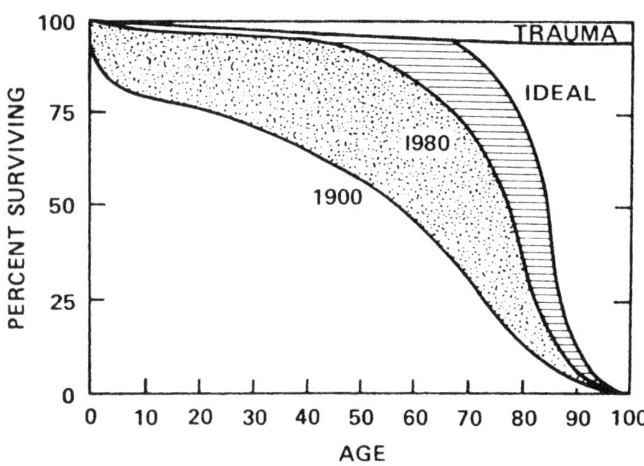

Fig. 1. Actual and projected survival curves for humans. The maximum life span here is assumed to be 100 years. As variables that cause death prior to reaching the age of the life span decrease, rectangularization of the survival curve occurs. As indicated by the stippled area, 80% of the difference between the 1900 survival curve and the ideal curve had been eliminated by 1980. Trauma is shown as the major cause of death in early life. (From Fries.[6] Reprinted with permission.)

Figure 1

with estimates ranging from 85 to 115 years.[3-5] In Fig. 1 the percentage of surviving patients is plotted against age. Note how improved survival of the population leads to a "rectangularization of the curve," as the elimination of premature death leads to an acute downslope at the value of the natural life span.[6] To achieve this rectangularization, good medical care and lifestyle interventions are essential.

Another result of the aging population is that a significant percentage of elderly patients will require surgical evaluation and intervention. In a review of 220,000 hospital discharges from 1972 and 1981, Valvona and Sloan[7] have shown that the rate of surgery among the elderly has increased markedly. Total surgical hospital discharges for patients aged 65 to 74 years increased by 93%, and surgical hospital discharges for patients aged 75 years or more increased by 123%. The largest increases were associated with hip arthroplasty, cataract surgery, and coronary bypass grafting. The incidence of common general surgical procedures has increased as well, with the exception of surgery for peptic ulcer disease (Table 1). The data for the elderly patients also showed a significant 20% to 30% drop in postoperative mortality. Valvona and Sloan concluded that "the surgical utilization has outpaced the growth of the number of surgeons with the result that the surgeons' workload has actually increased." Thus, general surgeons need to seriously address the increasing number of elderly patients requiring simple and complicated surgical care, and be prepared to meet their specific needs.

Table 1

A significant percentage of elderly patients will be debilitated, and many will be residents of nursing homes. A recent study calculated that as many as 43% of the 2.2 million people who turned 65 in 1990 can be expected to enter a nursing home before they die. Of this population, 32% will spend more than 3 months in a nursing home, 24% will spend more than 1 year in a nursing home, and 9% will spend more than 5 years in a nursing home.[8]

HISTORY

The first organized analyses of the risks of operating on the elderly appeared around the turn of the century. Prior to this the general consensus was that advanced age, per se, was an absolute contraindication to elective and emergency surgery. In 1907, Smith[9] reported on 165 patients over the age of 50 years who underwent surgery for hernias, appendicitis, and breast cancer, among other maladies. The overall mortality was 19%. He stressed that "because [the patients] are old, we must not consider that it is time for them to die ... we should endeavor to prolong life, and prolong it in comfort." He also stressed the appropriateness of "surgical interference in emergencies which threaten life and in conditions which destroy the peace and comfort of the elderly."

Changing attitudes concerning surgery in the elderly

In 1937, Brooks[10] reported on 293 patients over the age of 70 years who underwent surgery. He emphasized the importance and benefit of operative procedures performed exclusively for the relief of distressing symptoms.

In 1961, Wilder and Fishbein[11] reported on 207 patients over the age of 80 years who underwent surgery. The authors noted that excellent results could be obtained even in acutely ill patients. They concluded that "the postponement of elective procedures in elderly patients, either free of significant concomitant disease or not, is often unwise," since conversion to an emergency operation carries a higher morbidity and mortality.

Table 1. Surgical Trends, 1972–1981

	1972 Patient Age (yr)		1981 Patient Age (yr)	
	65–74	>75	65–74	>75
Procedure	Number of Procedures Performed (in 1,000s)			
Coronary artery bypass grafting	2.5	8.0	46.0	6.8
Rectal cancer surgery	5.2	4.7	11.8	7.8
Endarterectomy	7.3	8.4	49.1	29.1
Cholecystectomy	63.2	29.7	84.9	52.8
Mastectomy	17.5	12.8	24.2	17.9
Vessel resection	8.2	3.2	8.2	6.1
Peptic ulcer surgery	31.2	16.9	23.8	21.8

Adapted from Valvona and Sloan.[7]

Table 2. Mortality Associated With Intra-Abdominal and Extra-Abdominal Procedures in Octogenarians, 1964

Intra-Abdominal Procedures	
Procedure	Mortality (Overall, 28.7%)
Colon surgery	30%
Stomach surgery	39%
Biliary surgery	7%
Small-bowel surgery	15%
Miscellaneous (gynecologic surgery, exploratory laparotomy, appendectomy)	38%

Extra-Abdominal Procedures	
Procedure	Mortality (Overall, 16.4%)
Hip arthroplasty	20%
Genitourinary surgery	12%
Amputation	20%
Herniorrhaphy	5%
Miscellaneous (neck, breast, peripheral vascular surgery)	20%

Adapted from Marshall and Fahey.[12]

Table 2

In 1963, Marshall and Fahey[12] reported the results of 120 intra-abdominal (alimentary tract and gynecologic) and 380 extra-abdominal (urologic, orthopaedic, herniorrhaphic, peripheral vascular, breast, head, and neck) procedures in 443 patients over the age of 80 years (Table 2).The authors concluded that intra-peritoneal operations were significantly more hazardous than extraperitoneal operations, and that perioperative morbidity and mortality could be minimized with aggressive pulmonary support. They also stressed that the risks were not prohibitive, and that emergency and elective procedures should be undertaken as necessary.

Improvements contribute to survival

Improved survival following the surgical treatment of octogenarians was documented in 1979 by Djokovic and Hedley-White,[13] who reported on 500 patients who underwent 664 surgical procedures between 1975 and 1977. The mortality was 6.2%. Major causes of death were myocardial infarction, gram-negative sepsis with pneumonia, and mesenteric ischemia. Recent improvements in perioperative anesthetic techniques, intensive cardiac monitoring, and prevention of pulmonary and systemic sepsis were believed to have contributed to the improved overall survival.

The effects of surgery on nonagenarians were first documented in 1972 by Denny and Denson,[14] who reviewed 272 patients who underwent 301 surgical procedures between 1958 and 1966. The overall mortality was 29%; patients without associated diseases had a mortality of 5%.

The first report of surgery in patients over the age of 100 years appeared in 1985 by Katlic.[15] Six patients underwent multiple procedures, including pacemaker implantation, herniorrhaphy, endoscopy, orthopedic surgery, amputation, and cholecystectomy. There was only one complication and no perioperative deaths.

It has become obvious that chronologic age is not a contraindication to surgery, and that quality surgical care can be critical in the optimization of the life span and rectangularization of the human survival curve (Fig. 1). In addition, active concomitant disease, especially of the cardiac, respiratory, immune, and renal systems, is an important determinant of patient outcome.

Realistic goals

As surgeons begin to treat more patients of advanced age, the need arises to define realistic expectations and goals. Maximization of life span should be paramount, but not at the cost of one's dignity. Curing disease is a righteous goal but, if this cannot be achieved, an aggressive approach to palliation and comfort should be just as important. A list of reasonable goals appears in Table 3.

Table 3

SPECIFIC CONSIDERATIONS

Age as a Risk Factor

Once physicians scrutinized the clinical course of elderly patients undergoing surgical intervention, chronologic age became a less important factor in survival than the condition of the patient's critical organ systems. These systems age at a defined rate and in a characteristic fashion.

Cardiovascular system

The Cardiovascular System. During and after surgical procedures in the elderly patient, stresses are placed on the cardiovascular system that can result in significant morbidity and mortality.

Anatomically, the cardiovascular system begins the aging process early.[16,17] Atherosclerotic plaque is present in the large blood vessels of as many as 30% of persons aged 15 to 24 years, and 85% of persons aged 35 to 44 years. Atherosclerosis also affects the coronary arterial system, with stenoses involving

Table 3. Goals of Medical and Surgical Care for the Elderly Patient

1. Maximization or maintenance of potential life span
2. Maintenance of dignity of life, maximization of self-esteem
3. Maximization of independent function, minimization of dependence
4. Relief of suffering, with particular attention to pain
5. Palliation and comfort

Adapted from Keating and Lubin.[2]

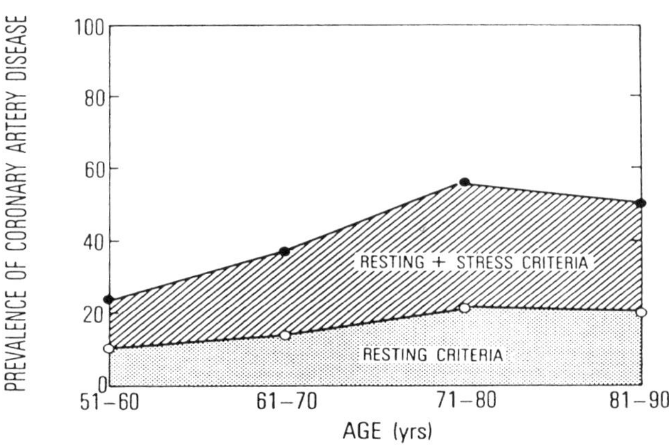

Fig. 2. Prevalence of ischemic coronary arterial disease in subjects enrolled in the Baltimore Longitudinal Study of Aging. Postmortem incidence of clinically significant coronary artery disease in patients over the age of 70 years is as high as 50%. Using routine resting cardiac criteria (defined as a history of coronary artery disease and abnormal electrocardiographic results), less than 50% of patients at risk were detected. When stress testing with thallium scintigraphy was added, additional disease was found, more in line with the autopsy data. (From Josephson and Lakatta.[17] Reprinted with permission.)

greater than 50% of the luminal diameter documented in up to 50% of people aged 55 to 64 years.

Age and the hyposympathetic state

In addition, the hormonal milieu of the cardiovascular system becomes altered. Aging creates a relative hyposympathetic state among the cardiovascular target organs. This is not due to a change in catecholamine levels, per se, but most likely to a decrease or defect in receptor response to catecholamines. This phenomenon has been documented in normal elderly subjects undergoing routine exercise. When exercising, both the young and the elderly increase cardiac output, but by markedly different mechanisms. Younger people increase heart rate and stroke volume by increasing the efficiency of myocardial contraction, as measured by decreased end-systolic volumes. On the other hand, older people exhibit minimal changes in heart rate but increase stroke volume by augmenting end-diastolic volume and moving up the Frank-Starling curve.

As a result of the hyposympathetic state, elderly patients respond differently than do younger patients to the intrinsic catecholamine augmentation induced by stress. This stress can result from surgery, hypovolemia, fluid shifts from third spacing in the postoperative period, and vasodilation and cardiac depression induced by anesthesia.

Figure 2

Coronary artery disease increases markedly with age, but much of it is not evident until after the stress of surgery. The Baltimore Longitudinal Study of Aging (BLSA) investigated the incidence of cardiac disease in the elderly population. Figure 2 illustrates the relationship between stress testing and coronary artery disease: the more intense the investigation, the more disease (and patients at risk for postoperative complications) will be found.[18] Hertzer et al[19] investigated a group of vascular surgical patients at highest risk for concomitant coronary artery disease by preoperative angiography, and found that 15% of patients without a clinical history of disease had surgically correctable lesions. In contrast, 44% of symptomatic patients had surgically correctable lesions when studied similarly. Preoperative evaluation of asymptomatic patients by dipyridamole-thallium imaging has also been shown to be superior to routine clinical assessment in detecting patients at risk.[20] Thus, much study has been focused on which elderly patients are at increased risk for cardiac complications after noncardiac surgery.

Overall, the cardiac complication rate (defined as the incidence of arrhythmia, infarction, congestive heart failure, and cardiac death) from general anesthesia and surgery is 0.2%. The presence of cardiac disease increases the risk substantially. During the 1980s better patient selection and advances in anesthesia and perioperative cardiac care resulted in lower morbidity and mortality. The morbidity rate has since been reported to be between 8% and 15% for patients undergoing surgery within 3 months of a myocardial infarction (decreased from 30% in the 1970s), and 3.5% for patients undergoing surgery within 3 to 6 months of a myocardial infarction (decreased from 5% to 15% in the 1970s).[21] Notable improvements in care include general medical status, arrhythmia therapy, hypertensive therapy, use of temporary and permanent pacemakers, Swan-Ganz catheter measurement of pulmonary artery pressure, and the appropriate use of inotropic agents.

During the past 16 years two major studies have addressed the issue of predicting cardiac risk in elderly patients undergoing noncardiac surgery. In 1977, Goldman et al[22] studied 1,001 such patients and established criteria that predict significant postoperative cardiac complications. Each criterion was given a point value based upon discriminant function coefficients (Table 4). Total point values greater than 26 (of 53) were associated with

Table 4

Table 4. Goldman's Criteria of Factors Predicting Cardiac Risk in Noncardiac Surgery

Factor	Statistical Significance*	Points†
S_3 gallop/JVD	$P<0.001$	11
Myocardial infarction within 6 months	$P<0.001$	10
Ectopy (non–sinus rhythm)	$P<0.001$	7
More than five premature ventricular contractions	$P<0.001$	7
Intraperitoneal, thoracic, or aortic procedure	$P<0.001$	3
Age above 70 years	$P=0.001$	5
Aortic stenosis	$P=0.007$	3
Emergency surgery	$P=0.007$	4
Poor medical condition	$P=0.027$	3

*Based on multivariate analysis.
†Based on discriminant analysis.
Adapted from Goldman et al.[22]

22% cardiac morbidity and greater than 50% mortality. Total values of 13 to 25 points were associated with 11% cardiac morbidity but only 2% mortality. The authors suggested that even patients in the latter group would benefit greatly from preoperative cardiac consultation, as 28 of the 53 points represent potentially controllable and reversible cardiac conditions.

In the other study, Gerson et al[23] showed, in 100 patients greater than 65 years of age, that the most predictive test for postoperative cardiac and pulmonary complications was a simple supine bicycle exercise. Patients who were able to exercise for 2 minutes and raise their heart rate above 99 beats per minute were six times less likely to experience cardiac complications, and five times less likely to experience postoperative major pulmonary complications than were patients who could not exercise.

Respiratory system

The Respiratory System. The elastic recoil of lung tissue lessens progressively with age, resulting in decreased compliance and increased closing volume. Compliance is further compromised as the chest wall stiffens. Diffusion capacity decreases as well, due to a decrease in the total functional surface area and an increase in alveolar-capillary membrane thickness. Finally, the respiratory muscles weaken in strength and endurance, and more dependence is placed on the accessory muscles of the abdomen.

Respiratory function is evaluated easily by routine pulmonary function tests and arterial blood gas analysis. Specialized tests can be employed as necessary. These include carbon monoxide absorption to assess alveolar diffusion capacity, nitrogen washout to assess uniformity of ventilation, and ventilation/perfusion analysis to identify the presence of pulmonary emboli and differential ventilation.

Identifying the elderly surgical patient at risk for pulmonary complications

Surgical intervention stresses the respiratory system; thus, it is imperative to identify patients at risk for pulmonary complications. Following laparotomy, vital capacity may decrease by up to 70%, and the respiratory drive may be depressed from the use of narcotics. In older patients, especially those with preexisting respiratory disease, postoperative atelectasis, pneumonia, aspiration, and pulmonary edema are common and potentially lethal. Gerson et al[24] reported a major pulmonary complication rate of 14% following abdominal and noncardiothoracic surgery in 177 patients over the age of 65 years. These complications included pneumonia, pulmonary edema, and pulmonary embolism. Atelectasis was not mentioned, but had it been included it most likely would have doubled the complication rate. There were three pulmonary deaths. Factors predictive of pulmonary complications included a forced expiratory volume in 1 second (FEV_1) of less than 45% of the predicted value, one or more Goldman cardiac criteria, and an inability to perform more than 2 minutes of supine bicycle exercise. Use of this simple screening test, or just identifying patients at risk by an inquisitive history (ie, asking them how far they can walk) can help identify patients at risk for pulmonary complications. Preoperative exercise and teaching, cessation of cigarette smoking, incentive spirometry, and medical optimization with bronchodilators are the only way to prevent these complications and increase the chance of successful surgical outcomes. Because postoperative pneumonia is associated with a 15% to 20% mortality in the aged, only early diagnosis and aggressive treatment with pulmonary toilet and empiric antibiotics can help reduce this figure.

Renal system

The Renal System. The aging of the renal system can be divided into two parts: glomerular senescence and tubular senescence.[25] Progressive sclerosis of the glomeruli occurs with normal aging, independent of the presence of such common diseases as hypertension, diabetes, and atherosclerosis. This aging pattern might be related to overall protein intake, which causes daily hyperfiltration and intraglomerular hypertension. Over a patient's lifetime this leads to progressive glomerulosclerosis and a loss of renal filtering ability, as measured by the glomerular filtration rate (GFR; ie, creatinine clearance). After the fourth decade of life, the GFR typically decreases by 1 mL/min per year.

Normal aging of the renal glomerular system is not detectable by routine laboratory tests, such as serum creatinine measurement. This is because of a concurrent loss of total body muscle mass and muscle creatinine production; thus, the serum creatinine level remains normal. However, creatinine clearance *in men* may be estimated from serum creatinine measurements using the following equation, which considers age as well as muscle mass[26]:

$$\text{Creatinine clearance (mL/min)} = \frac{[(140\text{–age}) \times \text{weight (kg)}]}{(72 \times \text{serum creatinine})}$$

To calculate creatinine clearance *in women*, the resulting value should be multiplied by 0.85 because of lower overall muscle mass. Normal creatinine clearance is 100 to 125 mL/min. Using this equation, a 40-year-old, 70-kg man with a serum creatinine level of 1 mg/dL would have a creatinine clearance of 97.2 mL/min, but an 80-year-old, 70-kg man with a serum creatinine level of 1 mg/dL would have a creatinine clearance of only 58.3 mL/min.

Along with glomerular senescence, the tubules age as well. Renal tubule length decreases, their basement membranes thicken, interstitial fibrosis develops, and atherosclerosis of the surrounding capillary bed occurs. This leads to a loss of effective secretion of solutes such as potassium and hydrogen, and resorption of solutes such as sodium.

The renal system at risk

The normal aging of the renal system places it at risk of injury due to ischemia and nephrotoxic drug therapy perioperatively. Perioperative injury is even more likely in the presence of other diseases that adversely affect the renal system (eg, diabetes, hypertension, glomerulonephritis, collagen-vascular disease, amyloidosis, urolithiasis, occult obstructive uropathy). However, such injury may be prevented by careful attention to the diagnosis and control of such conditions prior to surgery, and administration of the appropriate dosage of potentially nephrotoxic drugs and monitoring of fluid status before, during, and after surgery.

Immune system

The Immune System. As with the organ systems, the immune system changes with age.[27] These changes are subtle but ultimately can result in significantly altered responses to stress and infection by the elderly patient. Changes in immune surveillance also can result in the ineffective identification and destruction of tumor cells.

The solid organs of the lymphoid system (ie, liver, spleen, thymus) decrease in volume with age. The thymus, which is fairly large and cellular in the infant, is replaced completely by fat within 50 to 60 years. Cell-mediated immunity, the function of the T cells, also decreases with age. This is manifested by a decreased peripheral T-cell count, depressed proliferative response to lectins (eg, concanavalin A, phytohemagglutinin), a decreased mixed lymphocyte reaction, and a blunted cutaneous delayed hypersensitivity. The T cells produce less and respond less to stimulatory cytokines, such as interleukin-2 (IL-2), but are more responsive to inhibitory stimuli, such as prostaglandin E_2.

T cells

Similarly, there is senescence of the B cell, the mediator of humoral immunity. Although no change is seen in the number of peripheral blood B cells, there is a depressed antibody response to stimuli, both nonspecific (by pokeweed mitogen) and specific (through an antigen). These events have led geriatricians to vaccinate their patients against influenza, pneumococcus, and tetanus toxoid (booster) at a younger age. Evidence has shown that vaccination during the relatively young fifth and sixth decades is associated with a more effective antigen response than is vaccination during the seventh and eight decades.

B cells

Antigen presenting cells

Finally, the macrophage, a cell of the reticuloendothelial system responsible for phagocytosis and antigen presentation to other cells, also undergoes senescence. Although the former function does not change appreciably, mediation of antigen presentation is noticeably depressed. Production of the cytokine IL-1 is blunted in response to infection, thereby blunting T-cell activation. Interleukin-1 is also responsible for the generation of fever, and the blunted IL-1 production by the macrophage may be partly responsible for the blunted response to fever observed in the elderly. In addition, macrophages produce more prostaglandin E_2, which inhibits T cells.

There are numerous effects of immunologic senescence. First, there is an increased incidence of infection of the commonly colonized organs and the respiratory and urinary tracts. In addition, there is a decreased ability to defend the infection of areas such as the soft tissues, peritoneal cavity, and cardiac valves. Second, there is a less clear-cut clinical presentation of infection by fever, chills, cough, and urinary frequency than would be seen in younger patients. Third, there is depressed immune surveillance, a cell-mediated response to primary neoplasia and metastasis, possibly contributing to the well-documented increase in the incidence of cancer among the aging. To protect the geriatric population one must carefully screen patients, have a high index of suspicion, and even empirically administer antibiotics to patients with presumed sepsis.

Concomitant Disease

The presence of significant disease in the cardiac, respiratory, and renal systems markedly increases perioperative risk in the elderly. The presence of significant disease involving the central nervous system, manifested by dementia or stroke, or other active medical conditions (eg, cancer, diabetes, sepsis from a biliary source) are also important prognostic indicators. As the number of concomitant diseases increases, so does perioperative mortality. In fact, the American Society of Anesthesiologists (ASA) Physical Status Classification, which predicts surgical risk, does not use age as a factor, but predicts that patients with coexisting illness will have more perioperative difficulties than will patients who are otherwise healthy.

Figure 3

Many studies have shown that the risk of perioperative or anesthetic death increases with advancing age. In fact, this risk is most pronounced in the very young and the very old (Fig. 3). However, the presence of associated disease is clearly a more important factor for morbidity and mortality than is chronologic age. Tiret et al[28] showed that perioperative complication rates increased with the number of associated diseases among patients of various ages. It is also apparent that, when controlling for the number of associated diseases, morbidity and mortality from surgery is very low in the "young elderly" and only slightly higher in the "advanced aged" (Fig. 3). Failure to differentiate chronologic age and number of concomitant diseases easily can result in considering a patient too high a surgical risk for an operation solely because of his or her age, when appropriate treatment (palliative or curative) really could be performed with minimal risk.

Concomitant disease—a more important factor than age

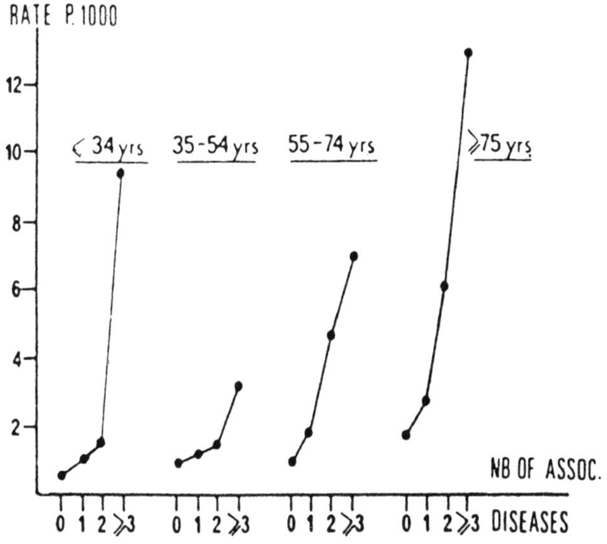

Fig. 3. Perioperative complication rates for different age groups, controlling for concomitant disease. Although an age-related increase in mortality is seen for patients with no associated illnesses, the difference is relatively small. Increasing the number of associated illnesses increases the mortality in all age groups, with the difference most pronounced at the extremes of age. Therefore, it is important to know where on the curve a patient undergoing surgery resides, in order to accurately estimate risk. (From Tiret et al.[28] Reprinted with permission.)

Emergency Surgery vs Elective Surgery

An important concept in surgical care of the elderly is the issue of emergency vs elective procedures. Numerous reports have documented that emergency procedures are associated with increased morbidity and mortality, and even the Goldman criteria give important point status to emergency surgery (Table 4). Similarly, Tiret et al[28] reported minimal differences in complication rates between emergency and elective surgery in patients whose ASA status was class I or II, but a threefold to fourfold increase in complication rates for emergency surgery in patients whose ASA status was class IV or V. Finally, in a series of 795 patients over the age of 90 years, Hosking et al[29] noted a 30-day mortality of 17.4% among patients who underwent emergency procedures, but only 6.8% among patients who underwent elective procedures. Serious perioperative morbidity (eg, myocardial infarction, pulmonary embolus, neurologic event, renal dysfunction, biliary dysfunction, prolonged mechanical ventilation) was also significantly higher among the patients who underwent emergency procedures than among those who underwent elective procedures (20.7% vs 7.5%).

Why emergency surgery carries an extra risk

Elderly patients are at higher risk of complications following emergency surgery because they seek medical help later, are diagnosed later, and are treated later than are younger patients. In addition, some surgical diseases might be more aggressive in the elderly than in the young. Due to the normal aging process, critical organ systems can be compromised following surgical intervention, and the acutely ill patient cannot fight the onslaught of complications as effectively. This is illustrated by two classic examples:

In a review of 104 patients with acute appendicitis, Lau et al[30] found a direct relationship between age and perforation rate: Patients aged 60 to 64 years had a perforation rate of 47% whereas patients aged over 85 years had a perforation rate of 100%. The overall perforation rate was 58%, morbidity was 24%, and mortality was 4%. Although the authors believed that appendiceal inflammation proceeded to perforation much more rapidly in the elderly (within 24 hours of symptom onset in 40% of patients), they were able to correlate perforation rate with delay in presentation to the hospital and delay in appropriate surgical therapy.

Timely recognition of surgical need is essential

In a review of 151 patients with gallstone disease, Houghton et al[31] reported a marked increase in emergency presentation among the aged, along with increased morbidity and mortality. Among patients aged 65 to 74 years, only 10% presented emergently whereas among patients aged over 74 years, 20% presented emergently. Emergency operations were associated with 66% morbidity and 19% mortality whereas elective cholecystectomy was associated with only 28% morbidity and 0.8% mortality. The authors concluded that because elective surgery is relatively safe and emergency surgery is so life-threatening, a more aggressive approach to symptomatic gallstone disease is appropriate.

These two examples highlight the need to aggressively approach the elderly patient with suspected surgical disease of the abdomen. Early referral for elective management of treatable disease, a high index of suspicion in patients who report abdominal pain, and early surgical intervention are paramount in ensuring a successful outcome and good quality of life for the patient. The advent of laparoscopic surgery, its application to all areas of the gastrointestinal tract, and the superb results reported thus far will help to reinforce this concept.

Withdrawal of Support and DNR Orders in the Operating Room

As medical care has improved and life expectancy has increased, our technical ability to maintain life by artificial means has become increasingly evident. This has given rise to the question of when to withdraw life-preserving support and has extended to the implementation and enforcement of "do not resuscitate" (DNR) orders.

Comfort, dignity, and the life-support option

In 1992 the American Medical Association published a report from its Council on Ethical and Judicial Affairs,[32] regarding decisions made near the end of life. That report stressed the need for attention to patient comfort and dignity (Table 3). The authors noted that there is "no ethical distinction between *withdrawing* and *withholding* life-sustaining treatment" (italics added), and that "the principle of patient autonomy requires that physicians must respect the decision to forego life-sustaining treatment of a patient." It is the physicians' "obligation to relieve pain and suffering and to promote the dignity and autonomy of the dying patient in their care ... [and to provide] effective palliative treatment even though it may foreseeably hasten death." Although the Council expressly prohibited physician-assisted suicide, it noted that adequate support and directed treatment toward relieving pain and suffering should diminish the demand for such intervention.

Deciding when to withhold or withdraw life support

Smedira et al[33] reported recently on 1,719 admissions to a medical-surgical intensive care unit (ICU). Life support was withheld or withdrawn from 7% of these patients. The decision to withhold or withdraw support typically originated during resident and attending work rounds, for reasons that included brain death, poor prognosis, futility of care, and extreme suffering. Although overall mortality was 12%, almost half (45%) of these deaths occurred in the ICU following withdrawal of support. Only 4% of the patients from whom support was withheld or withdrawn were considered competent; family members were involved in all of the other decisions. Almost all families ultimately supported physician recommendations, even those who disagreed initially. Among support withheld was vasopressor and antibiotic therapy, transfusions, infusions, and dialysis. The most humane withdrawal of support was felt to be the withdrawal of vasopressors first, and then mechanical ventilation. During withdrawal, sedatives and analgesics were given to patients as needed. The authors arrived at the following conclusions: (1) Although withholding and withdrawal of support occurs relatively infrequently, such decisions precipitate about half of all deaths in the ICU. (2) Because most patients were incompetent at the time of the decision to withdraw support, and most did not have advanced directives or living wills, open and frequent discussion with the families involved were tantamount to the successful implementation of the withdrawal. (3) Written DNR orders were very important because they led physicians and nurses to clarify the therapeutic goals for their patients, and basically were the critical decision-making points of their care. (4) The actual cost and allocation of critical care resources was never an issue in the decision-making process. It remains to be seen whether this will become an issue in the future (ie, whether there will be specific guidelines regarding the withholding or withdrawal of support).

The liberalization of DNR orders in the very ill and terminally ill has led to surgical consultations involving terminally ill patients for whom DNR orders are written. Indeed, some surgical consultants will not even evaluate patients following such an order, as they consider any care in this population to be futile. Is this attitude justified, and should these orders be honored in the operating room? Opinions often vary, depending upon the profession of the person giving the answer. Walker,[34] a medical ethicist, argued that DNR orders should be honored intraoperatively, and are not the result of our moral concerns about hastening patients' deaths from "correcting complications for which we feel responsible." He is of the opinion that deaths in the operating room should not be considered poor outcomes. On the other hand, Cohen[35] rendered a medicolegal opinion that DNR orders are not written in stone and, indeed, should be rescinded temporarily in the operating room and reinstated after surgery, all with the complete involvement of the patient and family. Following the publication of both of these reports a flurry of letters from surgeons and anesthesiologists argued emphatically that most respiratory and cardiac arrests or life-threatening events that occur in the operating room and during the immediate postoperative period are usually reversible. This includes hypotension due to spinal anesthesia and pulmonary edema due to third-space mobilization. They noted that resuscitation is much better controlled in the operating room than on the wards and has a higher degree of success in the operating room because the cause usually can be identified quickly and corrected. This clarification is a powerful argument for consciously suspending DNR orders during the perioperative period. This concept can be promulgated by educating the medical staff and the family of the patient prior to surgery. It is my practice to first council the patient and family regarding my plan, then suspend DNR orders prior to surgery. The orders are reinstated after 24 to 48 hours (sooner after minor procedures, later after major procedures). If a life-threatening complication occurs during the perioperative period, the patient is treated appropriately, the family is consulted, survivability is evaluated rapidly, and a plan is formulated quickly.

The pros and cons of DNR in the operating room

SURGERY IN THE NURSING HOME PATIENT

Complex surgical procedures can be performed in the aged population safely and expediently under elective conditions, and even in patients with concomitant diseases if these diseases are well controlled.

Geriatricians have implemented interventional services devoted specifically to care of the hospitalized and nursing home–bound elderly. These have been shown to increase quality of patient care as well as overall survival.[36,37] The geriatric assessment unit, a multidisciplinary unit providing medical, social, and rehabilitative care for the functionally impaired elderly who will eventually live in nursing homes, also has markedly improved independent function and decreased length of nursing home stay. Our clinical group believes strongly that a similarly structured service devoted to the *surgical* care of the chronically ill elderly in nursing homes will have a similar effect.

Geriatric Surgery Consult Service

Therefore, we developed the Geriatric Surgery Consult Service, whose goal is to improve surgical care to the frail elderly at home, in the hospital, and in the nursing home. This service is dedicated to the evaluation and treatment of general and vascular surgical problems in this patient population.

Accumulating experience

The Geriatric Surgery Consult Service was implemented in September 1991. From October 1991 through October 1992 we collected information on surgical consults involving 75 patients. Most (80%) were referred by the Johns Hopkins Geriatric Center; 96% came from nursing homes or were nursing home patients in our acute hospital. Mean age was 75 ± 2 years (range, 40 to 101

Table 5. Geriatric Surgery Consult Service: Categorization of Related Diseases and Medications

Related Disease	Patients (no.)*
Coronary artery disease	30
Hypertension	22
Neurologic disease	21
Diabetes	10
Vascular disease	8
Chronic obstructive pulmonary disease	6
Renal insufficiency	6
Postoperative infections	2
Cancer	4
Medication	**Patients (no.)***
Cardiovascular	26
Antiulcer	20
Antibiotics	14
Neurologic	9
Renal	3
Steroids	2
Chronic obstructive pulmonary disease	4
Thyroid	2
Feedings	2

*From a population of 75 patients.

Table 6. Geriatric Surgery Consult Service: Categorization of Patients by Number of Related Diseases and Medications

Related Diseases (no.)	Overall Frequency	Patients Undergoing Surgery	Patients Without Surgical Disease
0	24%	25%	21%
1	25%	23%	27%
2	24%	23%	24%
3	21%	25%	18%
4	3%	2%	3%
5	3%	—	6%
Medications (no.)	**Overall Frequency**	**Patients Undergoing Surgery**	**Patients Without Surgical Disease**
0	17%	20%	12%
1	33%	27%	39%
2	33%	34%	33%
3	14%	13%	15%
4	3%	5%	—

years; median, 74 years). Thirty patients were men and 45 patients were women. Eighty percent of the patients were considered "full codes," and 20% of the patients had active DNR orders. At the time of analysis, 53 were being followed actively; the remainder had died or been discharged from the facility. The average length of hospitalization at the time of consultation was 12.4 ± 3 months (range, 0 to 144 months; median, 7 months), and our mean follow-up after consultation was 115 ± 10 days (range, 0 to 337 days). Fifty-nine percent of the consults were urgent and 41% of the consults were elective. Of the admission diagnoses, 55% were for dementia or other neurologic disorders, 13% were for vascular diseases, 9% were for postoperative care, 4% were for chronic obstructive pulmonary disease, and 13% were for various other conditions, such as short gut or multiple sclerosis, or long-term placement. Of the referrals for consult, 23% were for maintenance (gastrostomy care, long-term intravenous care, or minor wound care), 20% were for abdominal complaints, 19% were for decubitus care, 15% were for help in determining a diagnosis, 14% were for vascular disease, and 9% were for breast examination. Table 5 lists the categorized related diseases and medications, and Table 6 categorizes the patients according to number of related diseases and medications. As expected, most patients had at least one concomitant disease, most commonly cardiovascular disease. Similarly, 66% of patients were taking at least one or two medications, most commonly cardiovascular preparations.

Table 5
Table 6

Of the 75 patients referred for surgical evaluation, 33 patients were deemed not to have an active surgical problem

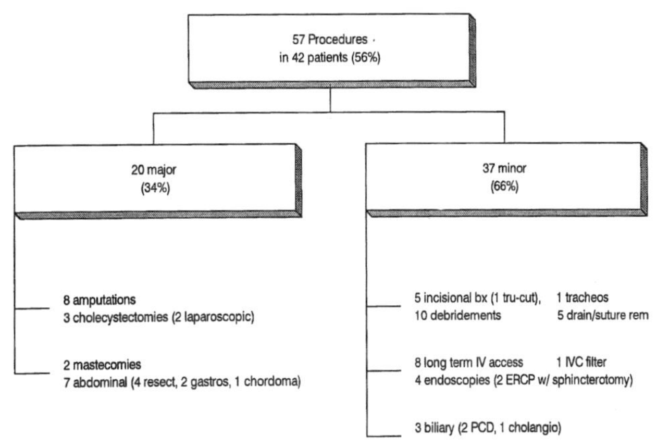

Fig. 4. Delineation of 57 procedures performed in 42 patients in the Geriatric Surgery Consult Service at The Johns Hopkins Hospital/Francis Scott Key Medical Center, Baltimore, Maryland. Surgical intervention was deemed necessary in 68% of the 75 patients; very few patients (or their families) refused treatment.

Figure 4

but were still followed. Forty-two patients (56%) underwent 57 total procedures (Fig. 4). Prior to all surgical intervention, DNR orders were rescinded temporarily and reinstated within 48 hours. Of the patients operated upon, 20 underwent major procedures and 36 underwent minor procedures. Debridement of chronic wounds, urgent limb amputation, and the establishment of long-term intravenous access were the most commonly performed procedures. Other common operations included surgery for breast carcinomas and gallstone disease, and intra-abdominal procedures.

Table 7

Table 7 lists the complications from surgical procedures in this population. The overall morbidity rate was 14%, and 30-day operative mortality was 2.3%. However, overall mortality was much higher, 21% (16 of 75 patients). Eleven patients who underwent procedures eventually died.

Table 7. Geriatric Surgery Consult Service: Procedures and Associated Complications

Procedure	Complication
Amputation	Death Colitis
Bowel resection	Myocardial infarction Sepsis/ventricular dependence
Endoscopy	Bleeding
Intravenous access	Vein thrombosis

Overal morbidity, 14%; overall mortality, 2.3%.

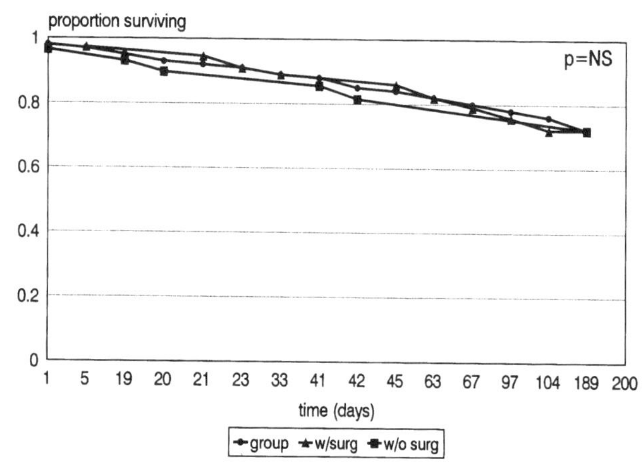

Fig. 5. Kaplan-Meier survival curves for the entire population of patients in the Geriatric Surgery Consult Service at The Johns Hopkins Hospital/Francis Scott Key Medical Center, Baltimore, Maryland, and the breakdown of the population between patients with surgical disease and patients without surgical disease. The overall 100-day survival was estimated to be 75%. No difference was noted between the curves.

Insights acquired through the Geriatric Sugery Consult Service

The prospective nature of this consult service has allowed us to identify and delineate the nature of surgical disease in this unique population and to compare data on demographics and survival between patients who required surgical intervention and patients who did not. There was no difference between the groups in number of concomitant diseases or medications (Table 6). Additionally, survival was equivalent among patients who underwent surgery, patients who did not undergo surgery, and the remainder of patients in the Geriatric Surgery Consult Service ($P = 0.4$; Fig. 5). Multivariate linear and logistic regression analysis showed that the number of related diseases and medications correlated with survival ($P < 0.05$), but not with the use of surgical intervention, type of surgery (ie, major vs minor; $P < 0.1$), duration of hospitalization ($P < 0.3$), or age ($P < 0.1$).

Figure 5

From our relatively small series one notes a number of important findings: (1) This is a frail population; the elderly are often afflicted with a multitude of concomitant diseases and take a number of medications. (2) Although wound care and maintenance are required in a significant portion of the geriatric population, many of these patients also develop common surgical diseases of the breast and biliary and abdominal systems. A number of limb amputations were performed but no major limb salvage procedures, because most patients were referred with very advanced disease. Most patients and families agreed to, and requested surgical intervention for lifesaving or palliative purposes; very few procedures (typically breast cancer surgery) were performed for cure. However, this referral population is obviously skewed, because attending staff did not refer patients who refused surgical evaluation. (3) Surgical procedures can be performed in this very frail population with very low complication and death rates. There were no intraoperative cardiac arrests or adverse events requiring emergency resuscitation. (4) There was no difference in survival between nursing home patients who require surgical intervention and nursing home patients who do not. Thus, one might infer that surgery in this population had no effect on patient survival. However, the majority of procedures performed were lifesaving (eg, amputation for infected limbs, gallbladder excision for acute cholecystitis) or life-maintaining (eg, long-term intravenous access for nutrition or antibiotics, wound debridement for the prevention of systemic infection, mastectomy)—surgery in these patients actually *improves* their survival. It may be concluded that while care in this population is not curative, it is not futile either. Quality of life, patient dignity, and relief of suffering take precedence over curative therapy.

ROLE OF THE GENERAL SURGEON

Typically, it is general surgeons who are cognizant of new techniques, such as laparoscopic surgery of the gallbladder, colon, and gastrointestinal tract; percutaneous drainage by interventional radiologists; and endoscopic procedures, such as percutaneous gastrostomy and laser treatment of malignant tumors. In this age of excellent anesthetic care and new surgical techniques, elective surgery is safe in the frail or advanced elderly. Toward this end, a specialized surgical service, run by a general surgeon, is critical to ensure the delivery of quality care to the nursing home elderly. We alone should be responsible for deciding if a patient is a candidate for palliative or curative surgery. Close collaboration with the anesthesiology team is paramount to ensure the safest anesthetic approach to even the simplest surgical problem. Educating patients, family members, and geriatricians about the roles and risks of surgical procedures, dealing with issues such as withholding or withdrawing support, and enforcing DNR orders in the operating room should be our responsibility.

The general surgeon as advocate

A case report in brief

As an example of our role in the care of patients toward the end of life, I will relate one brief case report. One of the patients referred to our Geriatric Surgery Consult Service was a 92-year-old arthritic woman with symptomatic gallstone disease that persisted for more than 1 year. She was receiving chronic antibiotics and pain medications for significant symptomatology after eating; her only other medication was a nonsteroidal anti-inflammatory agent for arthritis. Following evaluation by our service, elective removal of the gallbladder was recommended. This was performed laparoscopically without incident within 1 week of evaluation. The patient remained intubated overnight following surgery. After extubation, she was put on a diet and discharged to the Geriatric Center by postoperative day 2. Almost immediately thereafter she noted minimal symptoms after eating, and her appetite improved. She died from unrelated illness 3 months later. The patient, her family, her geriatrician, and the nurses caring for her felt that she was much more comfortable after removal of the inflamed gallbladder. Prior to evaluation the staff had believed that she was too old and frail even for elective surgery. Not only was she a good surgical candidate, but had a significant complication of the biliary system developed from the gallstones, I believe she would have developed sepsis and died shortly thereafter. This patient was helped by seemingly aggressive, but certainly appropriate surgical management. The patient, her family, and her health care providers needed to be educated about the benefits of elective surgery, as all were basically uninformed prior to the surgical consult. The patient's DNR order, in effect during her nursing home stay, needed to be rescinded during her procedure and the short time she spent in the ICU. Such a case brings to bear the utility of care of such patients and the need for such a specialized surgical service.

Trends in geriatric surgery consult service

Will such a consult service eventually develop into another surgical subspecialty? Surely precedent has been set with surgical fields such as pediatric and plastic surgery, and just as surely the expanding patient population will demand that someone take care of the geriatric surgical patient full-time. Some surgeons taking care of these patients will become recognized experts and be consulted frequently. However, the surgical problems faced by this unique patient population are fairly straightforward, and common or complicated wound care, the establishment and care of intravenous lines, breast disease, and alimentary tract disease could be handled easily by an aggressive, conscientious, well-trained general surgeon.

References

1. Vital Statistics Report. US Bureau of Census, 1980.
2. Keating HJ, Lubin MF. *Clin Geriatr Med* 1990;6:459-467.
3. Schneider EL, Reed JD. *N Engl J Med* 1985;312:1159-1165.
4. Barinaga M. *Science* 1992;254:936-938.
5. Schneider EL, Brody JA. *N Engl J Med* 1983;309:854-856.
6. Fries JF. *N Engl J Med* 1980;303:130-135.
7. Valvona J, Sloan F. *Health Affairs* 1985;4:108-119.
8. Kemper P, Murtaugh CM. *N Engl J Med* 1991;324:595-600.
9. Smith O. *Med Rec* 1907;72:642-644.
10. Brooks B. *Ann Surg* 1937;105:481-495.
11. Wilder RJ, Fishbein RH. *Surg Gynecol Obstet* 1961;113:205-211.
12. Marshall WH, Fahey PJ. *Arch Surg* 1964;88:896-904.
13. Djokovic JL, Hedley-White J. *JAMA* 1979;292:2301-2306.
14. Denny JL, Denson JS. *Geriatrics* 1972;27:115-118.
15. Katlic MR. *JAMA* 1985;253:3139-3141.
16. Lidman D. *Acta Chir Scand* 1982;148:575-580.
17. Josephson RA, Lakatta EG, in Katlic MR (ed). *Geriatric Surgery*, Baltimore, Md, Urban and Schwartzenberg, Inc, 1990, pp 63-74.
18. Gerstinblith G, et al. *Circulation* 1980;62(suppl III):III-308.
19. Hertzer NR, et al. *Ann Surg* 1984;199:223-233.
20. Boucher CA, et al. *N Engl J Med* 1985;312:389-394.
21. Goldman L. *Ann Surg* 1983;198:780-791.
22. Goldman L, et al. *N Engl J Med* 1977;297:845-850.
23. Gerson MC, et al. *Ann Intern Med* 1985;103:832-837.
24. Gerson MC, et al. *Am J Med* 1990;88:101-107.
25. Zawada ET, et al, in Katlic MR (ed). *Geriatric Surgery*, Baltimore, Md, Urban and Schwartzenberg, Inc, 1990, pp 85-96.

26. Cockcroft DW, Gault MN. *Nephron* 1976;16:31-41.
27. Powers DC, et al, in Katlic MR (ed). *Geriatric Surgery*, Baltimore, Md, Urban and Schwartzenberg, Inc, 1990, pp 173-181.
28. Tiret L, et al. *Can Anaesth Soc J* 1986;33:336-344.
29. Hosking MP, et al. 1989;261:1909-1915.
30. Lau WY, et al. *Surg Gynecol Obstet* 1985;161:157-160.
31. Houghton PWJ, et al. *Br J Sur* 1985;72:220-222.
32. Council on Ethical and Judicial Affairs. *JAMA* 1992;267:2229-2233.
33. Smedira NG, *et al. N Engl J Med* 1990;322:309-315.
34. Walker RM. *JAMA* 1991;266:2407-2412.
35. Cohen CB, Cohen PJ. *N Engl J Med* 1991;325:1879-1882.
36. Applegate WB, et al. *N Engl J Med* 1990;322:1572-1578.
37. Gracey DR, et al. *Mayo Clin Proc* 1992;67:131-136.

II Gastrointestinal Surgery in the Elderly

Ronnie A. Rosenthal, MD

BRIEF CONTENTS

BRIEF CONTENTS (continued)

INTRODUCTION

Table 1

The morphologic and functional abnormalities that accompany aging are responsible for an ever-increasing portion of the illnesses that confront the general surgeon today. Unfortunately, the early manifestations of these disorders tend to be subtle, and a major complication frequently is the first indication that a disorder is present. Therefore, we must learn to appreciate the subtleties in the presentation of these disorders in older persons in order to facilitate early diagnosis and treatment. The spectrum of age-related changes in digestive function is shown in Table 1.[1]

THE ESOPHAGUS

Physiologic Changes

The exact role of aging in altering the mechanics of swallowing has not been defined completely. Changes in the striated muscle involved in the oral and pharyngeal phases of swallowing have been observed with increasing age, but the role of these changes in disordered function is not clear. Alterations in the smooth muscle of the esophagus also have been identified, but the influence of these changes on esophageal motility is the subject of considerable controversy, and the etiology of the esophageal dilation found in the aged "presbyesophagus" remains to be delineated.

Swallowing disorders in the elderly

Regardless of the influence of physiologic aging, swallowing disorders are common in the elderly because of the increased prevalence of related pathologic processes. Degenerative neuromuscular disease, cerebrovascular events, disordered motility, and mechanical lesions can affect function at all levels. Surgical intervention may be necessary to correct many of these disorders.

Zenker's Diverticulum

Zenker's diverticulum is an outpouching of the esophageal mucosa and submucosa through an area of potential weakness in the upper esophageal sphincter. This area lies posterior between

Table 1. Age-Related Changes in Digestive Function

Oral Cavity		Small Intestine	
Mastication	↓	Transit time	(-)
Mandibular bone	↓	Motility/smooth muscle	↑
Salivary flow	↓(-)	Innervation	↑
Taste sensation	↓	Mucosa	?
		Absorption/enzyme activity	
Pharynx/Esophagus		Water/electrolytes	↓
Pharyngeal muscles	↓	Disaccharidases (lactase)	↓(-)
Esophageal motility	?	Fat	(-)
Gastroesophageal reflux	(-)	Fat-soluble vitamins	↑
		Water-soluble vitamins	(-)
Stomach		Vitamin D	↓
Gastric emptying	?	Folate/vitamin B_{12}	(-)
Acid production	↓	Protein	(-)
Pepsin production	?	Calcium	↓
Gastrin production	↑	Iron	↓
Gastric mucosa	↓(-)		
		Anus/Rectum	
Colon		Muscle wall elasticity	↓
Mucosa	↓	Continence	↓
Musculature	↓	Innervation	↓?
Transit	↓		

↓, Impaired or altered structure/function; ↑, Increased or improved structure/function; (-), no change; ?, uncertain.
Adapted from Nelson et al.[1]

Figure 1

the oblique thyropharyngeus and horizontal cricopharyngeus muscles (Fig. 1). As the diverticulum enlarges, it extends into the prevertebral space and may become large enough to appear as a mass in the neck. This pulsion diverticulum is thought to form as a result of increased intraesophageal pressure caused by a lack of coordination between pharyngeal contraction and cricopharyngeal relaxation, but there have been no convincing manometric data to support this hypothesis.

Small diverticula are best managed by simple cricopharyngeal myotomy. Dividing the cricopharyngeal muscle relieves the distal obstruction and allows the pouch to bulge freely through the incision, thus eliminating the neck of the sac. Resection, in addition to myotomy, is indicated for larger sacs. This usually is accomplished safely and quickly with a standard stapling device.

Achalasia

Achalasia, typically a disorder of the second to fourth decades of life, is found with increased frequency among the elderly.
It is characterized by elevated lower-esophageal sphincter pressure, failure of the sphincter to relax in response to swallowing, and an absence of peristalsis in the body of the esophagus.
These abnormalities are found in association with degenerative changes in the ganglia of Auerbach's plexus in the wall of the esophagus and, therefore, are thought to be neurogenic in origin.

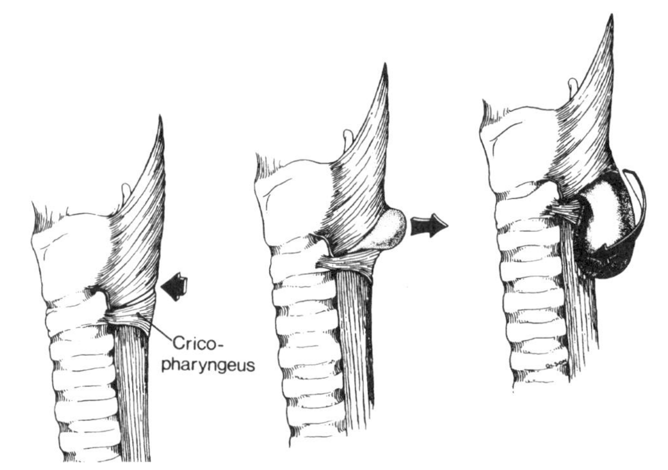

Fig. 1. Formation of Zenker's diverticulum. (Left and center) Herniation of the pharyngeal mucosa and submucosa occurs through a point of weakness at the junction between the oblique fibers of the thyropharyngeus muscle and the horizontal fibers of the cricopharyngeus muscle. (Right) As the diverticulum enlarges it dissects toward the left and downward into the superior mediastinum in the prevertebral space. (Adapted from Orringer MB, in Sabistan DC Jr [ed]. *Textbook of Surgery: The Physiological Basis of Modern Surgical Practice,* ed 14, Philadelphia, E.B. Saunders Co, 1991, pp 678-684.

Surgical procedures employed for achalasia

Achalasia is treated by esophageal dilatation or esophagomyotomy (Heller procedure). Pneumatic dilatation has been recommended in older patients because the interval of symptomatic relief appears to lengthen with increasing age, and the risks of complications and death appear to be lower than the risks associated with operative myotomy.[2] However, some authors have reported poor results of pneumatic dilatation and recommend myotomy for all but the highest-risk older patients.[3] The esophagus is approached through the left side of the chest and the myotomy is begun on the esophagus and carried down several centimeters onto the fundus of the stomach. To prevent gastroesophageal reflux (a common complication of operative myotomy), an anti-reflux procedure such as a Nissen or Belsey fundoplication is commonly performed.[4]

Gastroesophageal Reflux

When complications require surgery

Symptomatic gastroesophageal reflux is a common problem that is believed to increase in frequency after the age of 50 years. The two main mechanisms for control of reflux are a competent lower esophageal sphincter (LES) and effective clearing of refluxed gastric acid. Data regarding LES function in the healthy elderly have failed to show a correlation between decreasing pressure and age. Many drugs typically used by elderly patients (eg, nitrates, calcium channel blockers, anticholinergics, benzodiazepines) are capable of lowering LES pressure and promoting reflux.[5] The initial treatment of elderly patients with gastroesophageal reflux is similar to that of younger patients, and consists of lifestyle modifications and the administration of antacids, H_2-receptor antagonists, and promotility agents (eg, metoclopramide). In approximately 10% of cases symptoms will persist or a complication will develop in spite of adequate medical therapy, and surgery will become necessary. Peptic stricture, ulcerative esophagitis, hemorrhage, and mucosal metaplasia from squamous to columnar epithelium (Barrett's esophagus) are the most frequent complications requiring operation. Adenocarcinoma is estimated to occur in 8% to 15% of patients with Barrett's esophagus, necessitating surveillance as well as the prevention of further reflux. Stabilization and regression of Barrett's mucosa has been shown to occur once reflux is controlled by surgical means.[6]

Antireflux procedures, combined with dilatation when necessary, can be performed safely and with good results in most patients, regardless of age. In a series of 160 patients treated with the Hill posterior fixation procedure, 80% of those under age 60 years and 68% of those over age 60 years had good subjective and objective results. This difference was not statistically significant. In addition, 90% of patients treated early in the course of the disease had good results. Overall mortality was less than 2.5%.[7] Other series have reported similarly good results with the Nissen fundoplication in a number of patients, regardless of age.[8]

Cancer

Cancer of the esophagus is a disease of the elderly; it occurs most frequently in the seventh decade of life. Histologically, most esophageal cancers are squamous cell, although there has been an increased incidence of adenocarcinoma of the distal esophagus arising in Barrett's epithelium.

The preferred treatment for esophageal carcinoma is surgery when lesions are amenable to such therapy. Without resection, overall survival 1 year from diagnosis is only 18%. Recent data indicate that resectability rates are similar in younger and older patients (59%),[9,10] as are survival rates following resection (40% at 1 year, 22% at 5 years).[11]

Marginal pulmonary function may be a contraindication for resection

Postoperative mortality following esophageal resection for carcinoma is approximately 7% to 20% in the elderly and 3% to 14% in younger patients. This apparent increase in mortality, which has not been observed in all series,[12] has been shown to correlate with comorbid illness rather than with age alone.[13] Most complications and deaths are attributed to pulmonary causes in both age groups, and marginal pulmonary function may be considered an indication for palliation by bypass or laser ablation. Radiation therapy can provide effective relief of dysphagia in some patients with unresectable lesions, and has been used as an alternative to resection in patients with limited life expectancy or high operative risk.

THE STOMACH

Physiologic Changes

Age-related changes in gastric morphology, secretory function, and motility have been identified. There is a spectrum of alterations in the gastric mucosa, from gastritis to gastric atrophy to intestinal metaplasia (considered a premalignant lesion). The progression of gastric atrophy appears to occur proximally along the lesser curve of the stomach with increasing age. An increasing incidence of the antibody to *Helicobacter pylori*, as well as the organism itself, has been found in 50% and 80%, respectively, of patients over 60 years of age.[14,15] This correlates strongly with the presence of gastritis in the elderly, although its role as a causative factor has not been established completely.

H pylori

Mucosal changes also correlate with the decrease in basal and stimulated acid output shown to occur with aging. However, this correlation is not absolute; in one study as many as one third of patients with achlorhydria who were over the age of 80 years had normal mucosa.[16] Pepsin secretion also appears to decline, but it is unclear whether this is related to age, per se, or to alterations in the gastric mucosa. Serum gastrin levels have been shown to rise with increasing age, probably in response to declining acid output.

Mucosal and secretory changes

The gastric emptying of liquids slows with age whereas the emptying of solids appears to remain unchanged. The significance of this in the resting state may be minor, but delayed emptying can become a significant problem in the postoperative period (eg, following laparotomy). Altered emptying, particularly after partial gastrectomy, may lead to the development of bezoars.

Duodenal Ulcer

Duodenal ulcers are increasingly seen

Duodenal ulcer disease, previously thought to be a disease of midlife, is now seen with increasing frequency in the elderly. When duodenal ulcer disease does occur in this age group it tends to be virulent and associated with increased morbidity and mortality. Permutt and Cello[17] demonstrated a 15% mortality among hospitalized duodenal ulcer patients over 60 years of age compared with only a 2% mortality among patients under 60 years of age. Half of the deaths in the older patients were attributed directly to the ulcer disease. Statistics from the World Health Organization show that, in 1986, more than 80% of peptic ulcer deaths in the United States of America occurred in patients over the age of 65 years.[18]

Duodenal ulcers in the elderly may occur as an exacerbation of longstanding disease or as a new event. When the disease presents de novo, it tends to be insidious. An acute complication of the ulcer disease is the presenting finding in as many as half of older patients.

Nonsteroidal anti-inflammatory drugs (NSAIDs) have been implicated in the development of ulcer complications in the elderly.[19] In a report by Watson et al,[20] 40% of elderly patients with bleeding and 30% of elderly patients with perforation had been taking NSAIDs. Other studies have confirmed that older, rather than younger patients are particularly susceptible to the effects of these drugs.[21-24]

The atypical nature of the signs and symptoms of duodenal ulcer in the elderly often make the diagnosis obscure. Epigastric pain relieved by food or antacids is absent in nearly 35% of duodenal ulcer patients over the age of 60 years, but only 8% of patients between the age of 20 and 50 years.[25]

Table 2. Indications for Surgery for Duodenal Ulcer

Indication	Cutler[106] (1940–1945)	Kaplan et al[26] (1956–1969)	Watson et al[20] (1975–1980)	Permutt and Cello[17] (1977–1980)
Bleeding	23%	49%	40%	44%
Perforation	20%	16%	42%	50%
Obstruction	23%	24%	7%	6%
Intractability	34%	11%	12%	0%

Adapted from Permutt and Cello.[17]

The initial management of duodenal ulcers does not vary with age; however, a significantly higher percentage of older people will develop a complication of ulcer disease and require surgery. In the past, intractability and obstruction were significant indications for operative treatment. However, these indications have been nearly eliminated by the advent of H_2-antagonists and, more recently, the hydrogen-potassium adenosine triphosphatase (H^+–K^+ ATPase) inhibitors. Bleeding and perforation are now the two main indications for surgical management (Table 2).

Table 2

Bleeding duodenal ulcer

Bleeding is the initial symptom of duodenal ulcer in as many as half of the elderly patients in whom it occurs. Spontaneous cessation of hemorrhage is less likely in these patients, and recurrence is twice as frequent as in the young.[17] Death from bleeding is four to ten times more likely in older patients than in younger patients,[19] and surgery will be required to control hemorrhage in nearly 50% of the elderly.[20] Operative mortality correlates with the amount of blood transfused, and varies from about 7% for less than three units to 35% for five or more units.[26] Overall operative mortality varies from 10% to 18%; however, the mortality associated with nonoperative treatment is nearly twice as high.[20]

Attempts at endoscopic control of hemorrhage by sclerotherapy or bipolar electrocautery are warranted, but such treatment must be started promptly, monitored closely, and abandoned if control is not achieved quickly and completely.

Surgical treatment of bleeding

The surgical treatment of a bleeding duodenal ulcer is directed toward immediate control of the hemorrhage and long-term control of the ulcer diathesis. This may be accomplished by truncal vagotomy, pyloroplasty, and suture ligation of the bleeding vessel in 78% to 85% of cases.[18,21] Resection and truncal vagotomy is performed in approximately 15% of cases. This usually becomes necessary for technical reasons when the ulcers are large, and there is severe scarring of the duodenal bulb. The operative mortality for resection appears to be the same as or only slightly higher than that for pyloroplasty.

Perforation

Perforation is the most common indication for duodenal ulcer surgery in patients over the age of 65 years. Recent data from

England demonstrate a rise in the incidence of perforation, particularly among women.[27] The presentation of a perforated ulcer in the elderly is typical of the "atypical" signs and symptoms of acute abdominal emergencies in patients of this age group. Instead of the classic history of sudden onset of severe epigastric pain followed shortly by the development of a rigid abdomen, the elderly patient reports a prolonged history of vague abdominal discomfort, nausea, and vomiting. These symptoms may be so nonspecific that an abdominal catastrophe is not even considered. In one series, pain was not a significant complaint in 30% of elderly patients, there was no rigidity in 40% of elderly patients, and there was no guarding in 50% of elderly patients. In nearly 35% of these patients the symptom complex was so mild that they were thought to have medical rather than surgical illness.[28] Confirmation of the diagnosis of perforated ulcer in the elderly is made more difficult by the fact that, in 25% to 50% of cases, free intraperitoneal air cannot be demonstrated on standard upright chest x-rays.

There is little question that perforated duodenal ulcer requires surgical exploration and repair. Nonoperative management in the elderly is associated with mortality approaching 100%.[20,22] Normal inflammatory mechanisms that cause the omentum to migrate and seal off the perforation do not seem to function with advanced age. Continuing peritoneal soilage leads to overwhelming sepsis if surgical intervention is unduly delayed.

The choice of procedures is determined by the patient's general condition and the severity of the intra-abdominal sepsis found at surgery. Simple plication and omentopexy is indicated in frail patients with extensive inflammation. In stable patients with a long history of ulcer disease and minimal contamination it is desirable to try to control the ulcer disease in addition to repairing the perforation. In younger patients it has been demonstrated that the addition of parietal cell vagotomy to omentopexy decreases the chances of ulcer recurrence without significantly increasing operative risk.[29] However, patients over the age of 70 years were specifically excluded from these studies, and the addition of 1 or 2 hours of anesthesia may not be well tolerated by the older patients. Truncal vagotomy and pyloroplasty through the perforation is an alternative that can be accomplished quickly if the duodenum is pliable.

Operative mortality for perforated duodenal ulcers in older patients ranges from 21% to 32%, although rates as low as 11% have been reported.[30] The major determinant of mortality is the time from perforation to operation. Death rates have been shown to double when the preoperative delay extends beyond 12 hours.[31] There is also some suggestion that operative mortality is lowest following simple omentopexy, but the data are not conclusive.[26,31]

Gastric Ulcer

Although the majority of ulcers in older people occur in the duodenum, the majority of deaths from ulcer disease result from ulcers arising in the stomach. The incidence of gastric ulcers has

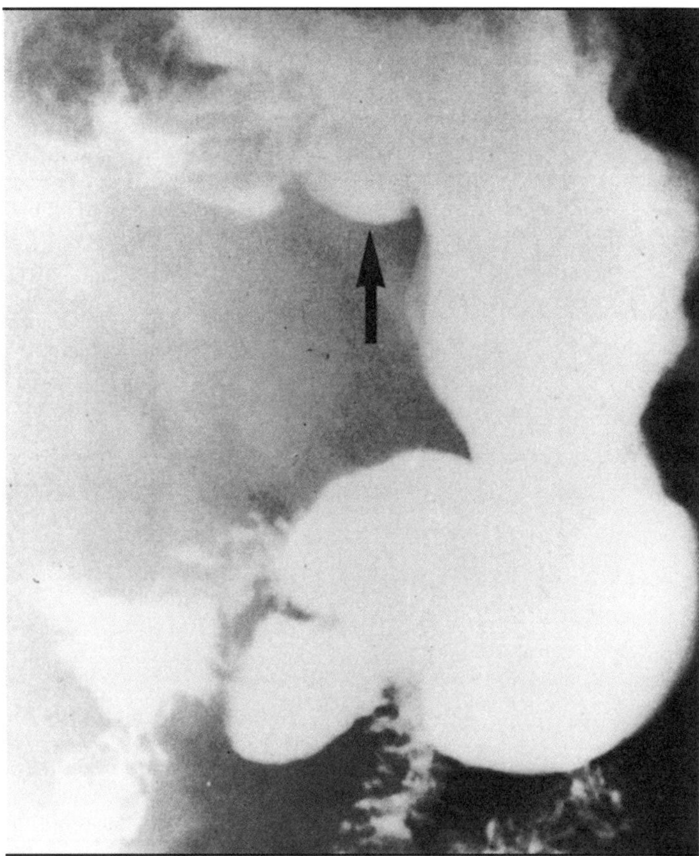

Fig. 2. Upper gastrointestinal series showing a large gastric ulcer high on the lesser curvature near the gastroesophageal junction. This ulcer has the typical appearance of a "geriatric ulcer." (From Amberg and Zboralske.[32] Reprinted with permission.)

increased among patients over 60 years of age. As with duodenal ulcer disease, the clinical presentation of gastric ulcer is often vague and misleading. Typically, gastirc ulcers occur along the lesser curve, at the junction between the antral and parietal cell mass. As the pyloric glands progress proximally along the lesser curve with increasing age, "geriatric" gastric ulcers often appear close to the esophagogastric junction (Fig. 2). The natural course of gastric ulcer disease is characterized by repeated episodes of exacerbation and healing. Until very recently gastric ulcer disease was viewed by most surgeons as a surgical disease. Prior to the advent of the H^+–K^+ ATPase inhibitors, recurrence rates following medical therapy were as high as 40% to 75%.[32,33] Recent enthusiasm for these inhibitors has led some to believe that the course of gastric ulcer disease will be altered.

Figure 2

Benign ulcers, when successfully treated medically, can be expected to heal by 50% at 3 weeks, 90% at 6 weeks, and 100% at 12 weeks. Repeated evaluation to monitor this healing is mandatory. Recurrence rates of 42% at 2 years have been reported in

Medical management vs surgery

patients whose ulcers heal within 12 weeks, and over 60% in patients whose ulcers heal more slowly.[34] Because gastric ulcers in elderly patients usually heal more slowly, such ulcers have an increased risk of recurrence.[32] Medical therapy is not completely satisfactory, as mortality as high as 40% has been reported among patients over age 70 who have been treated in this way.[35] Older patients who come to surgery as medical management failures will do so with complications; as many as 35% require emergency operations.[35] Elective operative mortality is only 2% to 9%, but mortality associated with emergency surgery is close to 30%.[30] Clearly, it is advantageous to be aggressive and treat these ulcers surgically before a complication occurs. Resection for intractability (failure to heal or recurrence) has been accomplished in elderly patients with operative mortality as low as 0%.[26]

Emergency gastric ulcer surgery

Bleeding and perforation are the major indications for emergency gastric ulcer surgery. When bleeding occurs it is frequently massive, and recurrent hemmorrhage is common. Initial blood loss severe enough to produce shock is probably the best predictor of continuing or recurrent hemorrhage. Death from a bleeding gastric ulcer is three times more likely than death from a bleeding duodenal ulcer. A short course of endoscopic coagulation is warranted but this approach should be abandoned early if hemorrhage is not controlled promptly. The mortality associated with the operative treatment of bleeding gastric ulcers is 14% to 26%.[26,30] Although this seems unacceptable, death rates for comparable medically treated patients are nearly twice as high.[36] Perforation is an even more ominous complication. In one series perforated gastric ulcer was associated with greater than 50% mortality whereas perforated duodenal ulcer was associated with only 11% mortality.[26]

The operation of choice for gastric ulcer is resection of the area at risk for ulcer development. Antrectomy to include the ulcer will eliminate the susceptible zone at the junction of the parietal cell mass. For ulcers high in the esophagogastric junction, a tongue of the lesser curve with the ulcer should be included. Vagotomy is not necessary unless there is evidence of duodenal ulcer disease as well.

Bleeding ulcers that are high on the lesser curve where resection may be difficult or time-consuming can be managed by oversewing the bleeding vessel, truncal vagotomy, and pyloroplasty. This is also an acceptable alternative to resection in poor-risk or unstable patients.

The appropriate operation for perforated gastric ulcers depends on the overall condition of the patient and the amount of contamination. Procedures vary from major resection to local resection or biopsy and simple omentopexy.

Cancer

Gastric cancer has not declined

There has been a decrease in the incidence of gastric cancer among the general population of the United States of America; however, the incidence among the elderly has not declined. Sixty percent to 90% of cases occur in patients over the age of 60 years. Changes in the gastric mucosa found in the aged, such as chronic gastritis and achlorhydria, are frequently present in association with gastric carcinoma. The significance of this association is not clear, although it has been shown that the age-specific incidence of gastritis associated with *H pylori* is similar to that of gastric cancer in some populations.[37] Morphologically, the tumors in the aged tend to be ulcerative rather than diffuse, and are frequently well-differentiated.

The nonspecific nature of the symptoms of gastric malignancies, particularly in the elderly, make early detection infrequent. The obscure nature of the presentation is reflected in the stage of disease found at diagnosis. In a large Italian study of elderly patients, Coluccia et al[38] found that 60% had stage IV disease at the time of diagnosis whereas none had stage I disease. At the time of exploration only 50% of patients were found to have resectable tumors. In countries such as Japan, where there is a high incidence of gastric cancer, screening programs are well-established. There disease stage at the time of diagnosis is lower, with approximately 50% of the tumors in elderly patients found to be stage I or II.[39] Surgical resection offers the only chance for cure and is often the best form of palliation for adenocarcinoma of the stomach, almost regardless of patient age. The extent of resection is determined by the stage and location of the tumor, not by the age of the patient. Operative mortality associated with curative surgery does not vary with the extent of the resection. Radical total gastrectomy, even with thoracotomy, is recommended in patients over 70 years of age if the chance of cure is good and there is little coexisting impairment. The mortality for total gastrectomy in the elderly varies from 3.3% to 12.2%, not significantly different from that in younger patients. The mortality for partial gastrectomy in the elderly varies from 2.3% to 10.5%. However, younger patients appear to tolerate partial gastrectomy better.[38-40]

Appropriate surgical procedures

Partial resection for palliation of bleeding or obstruction in the elderly can be accomplished with acceptably low morbidity and mortality. Total gastrectomy for palliation in this age group is not advised, and alternate methods, including laser therapy, should be considered.

Long-term survival following curative resection for gastric cancer is not a function of age. Coluccia et al[38] reported a 5-year survival rate of 23% among older patients but only 11% among younger patients. In addition, several older patients with stage IV disease survived for more than 5 years whereas no younger patient with stage IV disease was alive at 3 years. In Japan, where earlier detection has led to improved survival, 48.6% of older patients and 49.4% of younger patients are alive 5 years after curative total gastrectomy.[39]

THE SMALL BOWEL

Physiologic Changes

The small bowel undergoes relatively few changes of major clinical significance with age. Motility studies in humans indicate that transit time is unchanged, but motility in response to feeding may be reduced, suggesting a decline in the neurohormonal response to food. The only significant alteration in

Physiologic changes are minor

Table 3. Causes of Small-Bowel Obstruction

Age	Green[44] (1969) >65 yr	Zadeh[42] (1988) >70 yr	Mucha[43] (1987) 9–95 yr
Adhesions	39%	51%	49%
Neoplasm	3%	26%	16%
Miscellaneous	6%	19%	20%
Hernia	53%	4%	15%
Inguinal	54%		26%
Femoral	25%		9%
Incisional	7%		21%
Umbilical	9%		8%
Internal	5%	100%	28%
Other			8%

absorption is decrease in calcium uptake. This is thought to be due either to a decline in the production of 1,25-hydroxycholecalciferol by the kidney or a decrease in the amount or sensitivity of calcium-binding proteins in the mucosa.[41] The major surgical problems of the small bowel in the elderly are caused primarily by mechanical derangments and disease rather than physiologic alterations.

Obstruction

Table 3

Although small-bowel obstruction (SBO) is a major cause of emergency surgical intervention in the elderly, there is a paucity of *recent* data regarding the etiology, treatment, and outcome of this disorder in this age group. Studies from more than 25 years ago showed that just over 50% of SBOs in older patients were caused by incarcerated abdominal wall hernias; another 40% were a result of postoperative adhesions (Table 3).[42-44] Recently Zadeh et al[42] reported that adhesions now account for over half of the obstructions in the elderly; external hernia was not mentioned in this report. Instead, neoplasms have become more common and now account for over one quarter of obstructions. In a larger series of SBOs in all age groups, adhesions were responsible for 49% of obstructions, neoplasms accounted for 16% of obstructions, and hernias were responsible for only 15% of obstructions.[43] The incidence of hernias in the elderly population has not declined in the past 25 years. These shifts in the etiology of SBO may indicate that elective repair of hernias is becoming more widely excepted, even in older patients.

Adhesions

Extrinsic Causes. Postoperative adhesions account for approximately 80% of adhesive SBOs. Colonic, gynecologic, and other pelvic operations are probably responsible for the majority of adhesive SBOs in the elderly. Elderly patients with chronic partial obstruction often are malnourished from months of avoiding the symptoms associated with eating. The presence of cachexia in these patients may be mistaken for a sign of occult malignancy. The remaining 20% of adhesions are inflammatory. These can be primary, from infections such as tuberculosis, old pelvic inflammatory disease, and primary bacterial peritonitis, or secondary to intra-abdominal abscess from perforation of the appendix, a diverticulum, or foreign body. The systemic signs of these infections are frequently so subtle that the diagnosis is not made until the SBO develops.

Difficult to diagnose

The management of SBO depends on the completeness of the obstruction and the risk of strangulation. Partial adhesive SBOs, particularly those that occur during the immediate postoperative period, will resolve with nasogastric decompression in 51% to 88% of cases, with minimum risk of strangulation.[45] On the other hand, complete obstruction will require surgery in over 67% of cases. Unfortunately, there are no accurate markers of strangulation, particularly in elderly patients. Physical findings are notoriously misleading. Therefore, it is most important to avoid the temptation to manage complete obstruction in older patients with prolonged nonoperative therapy. Strangulation requiring resection will have occurred by the time surgery is performed in approximately 50% of elderly patients with adhesive SBO.[42,44]

Bowel obstruction secondary to hernia

Abdominal wall hernias occur in 13 of every 1,000 men over 65 years of age; the incidence in women is one fourth to one eighth that in men.[46] In the past, 15% to 30% of hernia repairs in the elderly were undertaken as emergencies for incarceration and bowel obstruction. More recently the incidence of emergency procedures has fallen to less than 20%, although emergency repair is still required four times more frequently in patients over the age of 65 years than in those under the age of 65 years.[47] Indirect inguinal hernias in men and femoral hernias in women are the most likely to incarcerate. Umbilical and ventral hernias each account for approximately 10% of cases. The duration of symptoms from bowel obstruction secondary to hernia is usually shorter than that for adhesive obstruction. In spite of this, strangulation requiring small-bowel resection occurs in nearly 30% of cases.[43] There are no controversies in the timing of treatment of incarcerated abdominal wall hernias; immediate resuscitation and operation are indicated.

Internal hernias are far less common than external abdominal wall hernias, and account for about 5% of obstructions.[42] Most of these hernias occur through mesenteric defects made during a previous operation and are difficult to distinguish from adhesive obstruction.

Figure 3

An uncommon but most insidious cause of SBO is herniation through a defect in the obturator canal (Fig. 3). This obturator hernia usually occurs in frail elderly women, and is thought to be caused by relaxation of the pelvic musculature with aging and parity combined with decreased loss of extraperitoneal fat and increased intra-abdominal pressure. The lack of external signs often makes diagnosis difficult. Preoperative delays of several days are common. The diagnosis is not established until the time of surgery in about two thirds of cases, and strangulation is present in over half of cases.[48]

Metastatic disease to the peritoneal cavity, which may be extrinsic or intrinsic to the bowel wall, causes a particularly difficult form of SBO. The symptoms usually develop over a

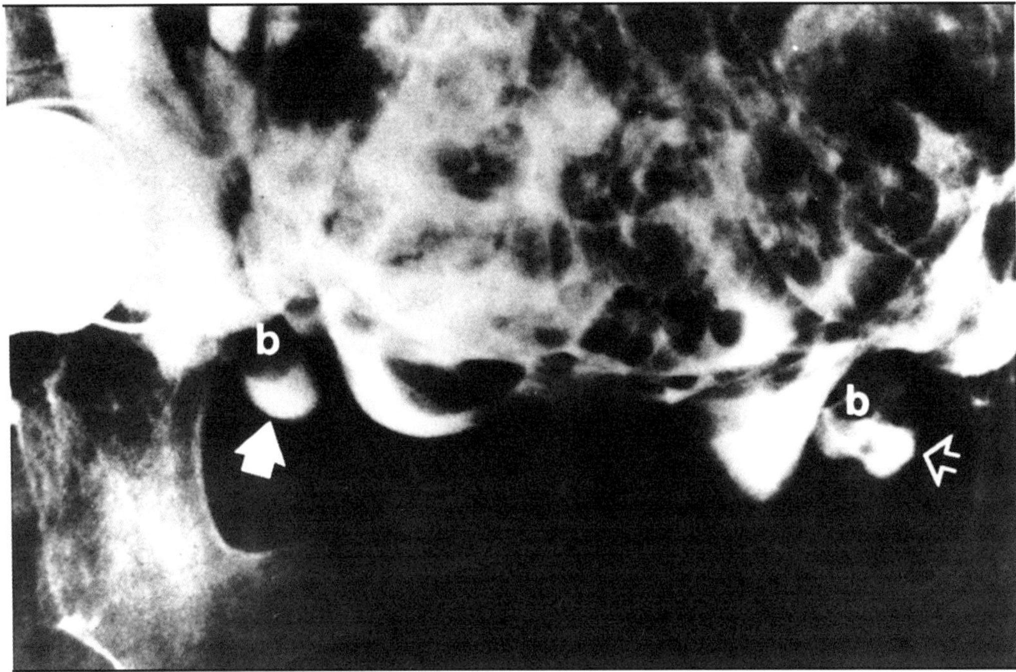

Fig. 3. Herniography demonstrating intraperitoneal contrast agent in bilateral obturator hernia sacs (arrows). (From Persson NH, et al. *Acta Chir Scand* 1987;153:361-364. Reprinted with permission.)

Metastatic disease

period of several weeks, but may be present for as long as 6 months. Colon, pancreatic, gastric, and gynecologic malignancies are the usual sources of this kind of obstruction, although metastatic disease from breast cancer, melanoma, and lung cancer also can cause obstruction.

This form of obstruction is difficult from a technical and ethical standpoint. Often metastatic obstruction occurs at more than one location in the bowel. Resection is frequently not feasible. Bypass of long, particularly obstructed segments may be possible technically, but can result in a functional short gut. Over one third of elderly patients with this form of obstruction die within 30 days of operation,[42] and the majority of patients are dead at 6 months.[43] This dismal outcome has led some to advocate prolonged periods of nonoperative decompression, but this produces only transient relief of the obstructive symptoms. In addition, the presence of a prior malignancy does not necessarily indicate that the obstruction is due to metastatic disease. A benign cause is found at the time of operation in approximately 10% to 38% of patients with suspected malignant obstruction.[45]

Criteria for surgical management

Therefore, management should be determined by the same criteria used for other forms of SBO. Negative indications for surgery should include short life expectancy and prohibitive operative risk rather than the presence of malignancy.

Intrinsic Causes. Primary neoplasms of the small bowel are very uncommon; the incidence of benign lesions is only 0.1% to 0.8%. Adenomas, leiomyomas, and lipomas are the most common benign tumors. Occasionally they may cause obstruction by serving as the lead point for an intussusception, but usually are incidental findings at autopsy.

Adenocarcinoma and carcinoid tumors

The incidence of malignant tumors of the small bowel is even lower than that of benign tumors, but the majority of symptomatic lesions are malignant. These tumors account for approximately 2% of all gastrointestinal (GI) cancers. Adenocarcinoma and carcinoid tumors are the two most common malignant neoplasms, and have a peak incidence in the fifth and sixth decades of life; however, they can occur in the elderly as well. Both tumors may produce symptoms of partial SBO that go unrecognized for many months. Metastatic disease is present at the time of exploration in over 50% of patients with adenocarcinoma; 5-year survival is only 20% to 25%.[49] In patients with carcinoid tumors the presence of metastasis is determined by the size of the tumor. In 80% of tumors larger than 2 cm, metastasis will be present at the time of diagnosis. However, 5-year survival is better, approaching 54%.[50]

Crohn's disease and SBO

Inflammatory lesions are an infrequent cause of SBOs in the elderly but deserve mention because they are rarely considered in the differential diagnosis in this age group. Obstruction secondary to Crohn's disease is similar in younger and older patients. Acute obstruction will usually resolve with bowel rest and appropriate medical therapy, but surgical intervention for more chronic obstruction is common.

Radiation and SBO

Radiation-induced strictures also can be considered inflammatory lesions. Elderly patients, particlarly those with underlying atherosclerosis, hypertension, or diabetes mellitus, or a history of surgery, are at increased risk for radiation injury. The surgical treatment for radiation-induced SBO is fraught with complications and should be avoided if at all possible. However, the operative morbidity and mortality associated with bypass is considerably lower than that associated with resection; thus, bypass is preferred in most cases.[51]

Luminal Obturation. Concretions of various ingested materials that usually form inside the stomach can migrate into the small bowel, producing obstruction. Phytobezoars are composed of poorly digested fruit and vegetable matter. These concretions form most frequently in patients who have undergone gastric resection but can also occur in older patients with intact GI tracts. Gastric stasis, high-fiber diets, and poor dentition are thought to be responsible for their formation in the latter group.[52] Bezoars can be removed from the stomach by commercially available enzyme products and endoscopic extraction, but once they have entered the small bowel, surgery is usually necessary. At operation the fibrous material can be seen as a boggy mass with dilated bowel proximal and collapsed bowel distal. Occasionally, the mass can be disrupted manually through the intact bowel wall and the contents milked through the ileocecal valve, but enterotomy with removal of the concretion is usually the safest way of avoiding recurrent obstruction.

Bezoars and SBO

Gallstone ileus is responsible for 1% to 3% of all cases of SBO, but has been implicated in as many as 25% of cases in patients over 65 years of age who have not undergone surgery previously. (Details of the presentation and controversies in the management may be found in the section *Hepatobiliary and Pancreatic Disease in the Elderly*, p 55.)

Inflammatory Bowel Disease

Although inflammatory bowel disease (IBD) is typically a disease of youth, a second peak of incidence has been noted near the age of 70 years, with the elderly comprising approximately 10% of all patients with this disorder. In younger and older patients, ulcerative colitis occurs up to three times as frequently as Crohn's disease. Yet, despite the fact that the clinical characteristics of IBD are similar in the young and old, it is initially recognized in more than 95% of younger patients but less than 67% of older patients.[53]

Ulcerative colitis

Ulcerative colitis in the elderly is confined with increasing frequency to the rectosigmoid. Although the disease tends to be less extensive, the first attack is more often severe, with mortality in the aged more than double that in the young.[54] Toxic megacolon and perforation without toxic dilatation also occur with increased frequency in older patients. Early surgical intervention for megacolon has been suggested as a possible means of keeping mortality low, but there are no data to confirm the utility of this approach. In older patients the response of ulcerative colitis to medical therapy appears to be good, although some studies report an increased need for systemic steroids with advanced age.[53] Remission can be achieved in most older patients; only 8% require operation.[56] Relapse occurs less often than in younger patients, and long-term survival is similar to what would be expected in elderly patients without disease.[57]

Crohn's disease

Like ulcerative colitis, Crohn's disease tends to occur more distally in older patients. In over 50% of cases the disease is confined to the colon, particularly the left colon in older women. Older patients present more frequently with hematochezia and are found to have a higher incidence of associated cardiovascular and diverticular disease. Pain is a less common complaint, and palpable abdominal masses are present less often. When the disease is confined to the colon in this age group the response to medical management is fairly good, with only 25% of patients requiring operation.[56] Patients with colonic Crohn's disease require operative intervention less frequently than do those with ileocecal Crohn's disease, regardless of age. Obstruction and perforation with abscess and fistula are the two most common indications for surgery. In spite of the need for resection in as many as 75% of older patients with ileal Crohn's disease, the outcome is usually good.[58] Operative mortality does not increase with advancing age, and the long-term prognosis is at least as good as, if not better than that for patients with early-onset disease.

Acute Mesenteric Ischemia

This is an abdominal disaster associated with a 50% to 80% mortality. Direct occlusion of the superior mesenteric artery by embolus or thrombosis and nonocclusive splanchnic vasoconstriction secondary to hypoperfusion are the major causes of this extremely lethal bowel injury. With recent advances in

Emboli

hemodynamic monitoring and management, the portion of ischemic events caused by low flow–induced vasoconstriction has declined, and emboli to the superior mesenteric artery are now responsible for over 50% of cases.[59]

Some improvement in the outcome of this devastating injury can be seen when an aggressive approach to diagnosis and therapy is used. Boley et al[60] have identified clinical characteristics that place patients at increased risk for ischemic events. These include age over 50 years with valvular or atherosclerotic cardiac disease, cardiac arrhythmias, recent myocardial infarction, intractable congestive heart failure, and hypovolemia and hypotension of any etiology. Patients taking medications that cause splanchnic vasoconstriction (eg, digitalis) also are considered to be at increased risk. Boley initiated a diagnostic and therapeutic protocol in patients at risk who developed acute abdominal pain out of proportion to their physical findings. The most essential part of the protocol was immediate arteriography. This was followed by surgery for occlusive ischemia or continuous infusion of vasodilating drugs via the angiography catheter for nonocclusive ischemia. The survival rate of 54% reported in this study is considerably better than that of most other series. In addition, survival was reported in ten of the 11 patients who did not have peritoneal signs at the time of initial evaluation.

Factors that place patients at risk for mesenteric ischemia

At operation for acute mesenteric ischemia the amount and degree of compromised bowel is often difficult to assess. If revascularization is indicated, areas of irreversible ischemia must be sought following reperfusion. Fluorescein perfusion and Doppler flow determination have been used to assess viability, but neither has been totally satisfactory. Clinical judgment and minimum resection with planned second-look surgery at 24 hours are still the most successful means of limiting tissue loss and preventing unnecessary morbidity.

THE COLON

Physiologic Changes

Some age-related changes in morphology and motility of the colon have been identified, but their correlation with functional alterations in the proximal colon is not well defined. There is atrophy of the mucosa, hypertrophy of the muscularis mucosa, atrophy of the muscularis externa, and an increase in the amount of connective tissue elements, but a loss in flexibility. In animals transit time increases with age, but in humans it appears not to change.

Significance of age-related changes

Age-related changes have a greater functional implication in the anorectal portion of the large bowel. With increasing age there is an increase in the diameter of the rectum, a decrease in resting anal pressure and maximal external sphincteric squeeze pressure, and a probable loss of anorectal canal elasticity. In addition, the rectal volume necessary to inhibit sphincter tone decreases, but the sensory response to rectal distention remains normal. In elderly women, functional impairment of the external anal sphincter and puborectalis muscles has been linked to pudenal nerve injury but the etiology of this damage is uncertain.

Fecal continence depends on a complex interaction of neuromuscular events. Any of the above changes may be sufficient to disrupt normal function and lead to the increased incidence of incontinence seen even in ambulatory older individuals.

Lower Gastrointestinal Bleeding

Diverticulosis and angiodysplasia

The two major causes of lower GI hemorrhage in the elderly are diverticulosis and angiodysplasia. Unfortunately, determining which is the source of bleeding can be difficult because angiodysplasia is found in over 25% of people in this age group,[61] and diverticula are found in nearly 50% of people in this age group. Angiodysplasia is a degenerative lesion that is nearly always found on the right side of the colon. Diverticula typically occur in the sigmoid colon; however, in older patients, hemorrhage from diverticula most often arises from the right colon as well.

Some insight into the source of hemorrhage can be gleaned from the pattern of bleeding. The source of a diverticular bleed is the perforating nutrient artery adjacent to the orifice of the pouch. The initial bleeding is arterial and usually quite massive. The hemorrhage ceases spontaneously in over 80% of cases, indicating that the offending artery has clotted. Rebleeding is not common. On the other hand, the source of bleeding from angiodysplasia is a dilated submucosal vein. The bleeding tends to be less severe initially, and also spots spontaneously. However, unlike the clotted artery of a diverticula, angiodysplasic lesions continue to progress until actual arteriovenous malformations develop. Recurrent bleeding occurs in approximately 80% of cases and will be more pronounced with each successive episode.

Although these patterns may suggest the bleeding source, accurate localization is essential, and a diagnostic workup must be started at once.

The best treatment for persistent, recurrent, or massive lower GI hemorrhage is selective resection of the portion of the colon that contains the bleeding site. Nearly all bleeding from angiodysplasic lesions and most diverticular bleeding is from the right side of the colon; therefore, right hemicolectomy will be required in the majority of cases. The presence of diverticulae on the left side of the colon in patients with a demonstrated right-side bleeding source is not an indication to extend the resection to a total abdominal colectomy. This procedure is rarely necessary if localization attempts have been aggressive, and is reserved for patients in whom no bleeding source has been found. The mortality for emergency total abdominal colectomy in the elderly ranges from 15% to 50%[62]; disabling diarrhea has been reported in nearly 15% of patients.[61,63]

Ischemic Colitis

Table 4

Colonic ischemia is the most common vascular disorder of the bowel. Ninety percent of patients are over the age of 60 years, and 95% of cases occur as isolated events. This disorder has a spectrum of presentations from reversible ischemic colitis to ischemic stricture to fulminant colonic necrosis. The possible causes of colonic ischemia are listed in Table 4, although no

Table 4. Causes of Colonic Ischemia

Inferior mesenteric artery thrombosis	Vasculitis
Arterial embolus	Strangulated hernia
Cholesterol emboli	Oral contraceptives
Cardiac arrhythmia	Polycythemia vera
Congestive heart failure	Parasitic infection
Shock	Volvulus
Ruptured ectopic pregnancy	Trauma
Digitalis toxicity	Iatrogenic
Collagen vascular disease	

Adapted from Reinus, et al.[64]

precipitating event can be identified in most cases. Approximately one in five cases is associated with another colonic lesion that may be causing partial obstruction.[64] Reversible ischemic colitis is the most common form of the disorder. The injury occurs in the sigmoid colon in 50% to 60% of cases. Submucosal hemorrhage develops early in the acute phase of the ischemia, and can be seen as "thumbprinting" on plain films or barium enema (Fig. 4). The diagnosis is established by sigmoidoscopy or colonoscopy. As the disorder progresses, early submucosal hemorrhages are replaced by ulceration. Subsequent complete healing occurs within 10 to 14 days in more than half of cases. Among the remainder, approximately one third progress to full-thickness infarction, one third form ischemic strictures, and one third develop a chronic colitis that is difficult to distinguish from IBD.[64]

Figure 4

The initial treatment for ischemic colitis is bowel rest and intravenous hydration; systemic antibiotics are reserved for more severe cases. Repeat radiographic monitoring for signs of

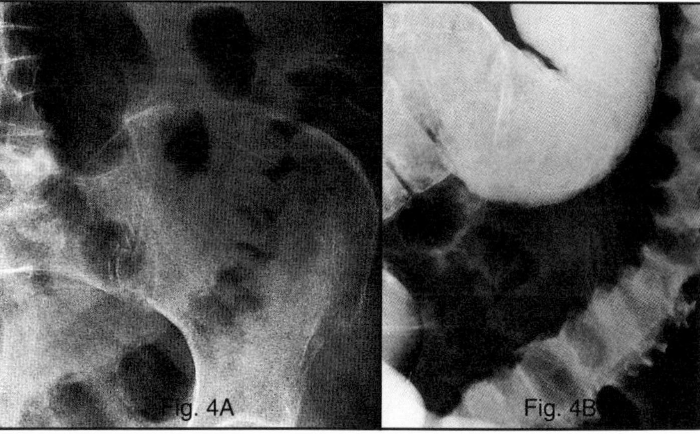

Fig. 4. **(A)** Plain film demonstrating "thumbprinting" of the sigmoid in ischemic colitis. **(B)** Barium enema in the same patient. (Courtesy of A. Gasparitis, MD, The University of Chicago.)

infarction or perforation is indicated. Caution must be exercised when relying on physical findings alone to determine the progression of the ischemia, as the signs of impending necrosis may be subtle in the elderly. Failure of hematochezia or diarrhea to resolve with several weeks of treatment is an indication that permanent damage has occurred. It also may indicate that stricture or chronic colitis will ensue, in which case resection is appropriate.

Diverticulitis

Although colonic diverticulae are present in over 50% of people in the ninth decade, only 10% to 20% of patients with diverticulae will develop symptoms or inflammation.[62] This inflammation is thought to be initiated by obstruction of a diverticula and subsequent perforation. This perforation may be microscopic and result in a pericolic inflammatory phlegmon, or it may be larger and result in a pericolic abscess. Free perforation is less likely, although rupture of a diverticular abscess with subsequent perforation may occur. The inflammatory process may erode into another organ (typically the bladder in men and the vagina in women), producing a fistula.

Differential diagnosis

The symptoms of diverticular inflammation in the elderly are often vague. Therefore, diverticulitis must always be considered in the differential diagnosis of elderly patients with vague abdominal complaints. The sequence of diagnostic studies usually begins with an abdominal flat film to look for signs of partial or complete obstruction, and localized inflammation, such as loss of the left abdominal fat strip or focal bowel dilatation. An upright chest film is necessary to rule out free intraperitoneal air. When an obstructive pattern is present, proctosigmoidoscopy should be performed first to include a rectal source of obstruction. When diverticulitis is suspected, insufflation with air during proctoscopy should be minimal. Most often, the proctoscope will not pass beyond 15 cm because of fixation of the sigmoid secondary to the diverticular inflammation. Colonoscopy during the acute inflammatory phase is not indicated. Abdominal and pelvic CT with triple contrast (ie, oral meglumine diatrizoate, rectal meglumine diatrizoate, and an intravenous agent) is the single best study to define the extent of the inflammation and the presence or absence of an abscess (Fig. 5). In the obstructed patient, a simple meglumine diatrizoate enema is sufficient to define the nature and site of occlusion.

Figure 5

Antibiotics and bowel rest

The treatment of diverticulitis varies with age. In the elderly, the signs of sepsis are often subtle and even a low-grade fever or slight leftward shift on differential should be sufficient to warrant hospitalization with intravenous antibiotics and bowel rest until the full extent of the inflammation can be evaluated by CT. With this regimen the majority of cases of diverticulitis will resolve without the need for emergency surgery. If the inflammatory process fails to resolve, operation becomes necessary. In this case, the procedure of choice is primary resection of the involved sigmoid colon with end colostomy and mucous fistula or, more frequently, closed rectal pouch (Hartmann's procedure). When primary resection is hazardous because of the extent of

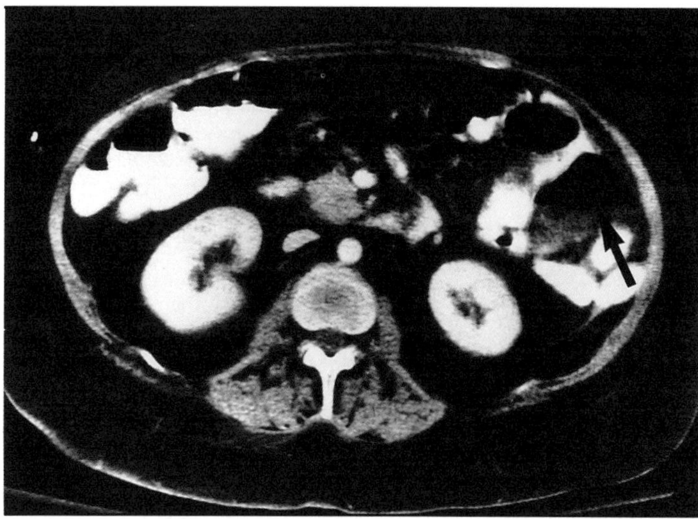

Fig. 5. Triple-contrast CT scan showing a large pericolic abscess in the left lower quadrant (arrow) typical of acute diverticulitis.

inflammation or the general condition of the patient, drainage of the abscess and proximal diverting colostomy is the procedure of choice. This is followed by resection once the inflammation has resolved.

Elective surgery

Indications for elective surgery for diverticular disease include repeat episodes of acute inflammation, fistulae to the bladder or other organs, stricture, and the presence of a deformity that cannot be distinguished from a colon carcinoma. Mortality for surgery in this setting is approximately 4%,[65] even in the most elderly patients. Emergency surgical mortality ranges from 17% to 30%.[65,66]

Appendicitis

In men past 80 years

Appendicitis, which is usually a disease of the second and third decades of life, is also seen with increased frequency in men over the age of 80 years. The disproportionately high mortality of 6% to 10% associated with appendicitis in older patients makes it particularly important to expect and recognize the atypical symptom complex in this age group.[67] The usual sequence of periumbilical pain followed by anorexia, nausea, vomiting, and localization of pain to the right lower quadrant at or near McBurney's point is uncommon in the elderly. Instead, there is a prolonged period of vague abdominal discomfort.

Early perforation of the appendix in the elderly has been attributed, in part, to pathophysiologic changes associated with aging. Narrowing of the lumen with fibrosis and fatty infiltration of the muscular walls can lead to increased pressure in the obstructed lumen. Atherosclerotic changes in the artery to the appendix are thought to result in a blood supply so marginal that even minimal increases in pressure lead to edema, vascular thrombosis, necrosis, and perforation. Perforation is found at the

Perforation

time of operation in approximately 70% of cases of appendicitis in the elderly, compared with only 20% of cases of appendicitis in young adults.[68]

Expeditious diagnosis and surgical correction are the prerequisites for good postoperative results. Nearly all deaths and most complications are associated with a longer history of symptoms and perforation at the time of surgery. A high index of suspicion and an awareness of the insidious nature of the presentation of this acute intra-abdominal inflammation in the elderly is necessary to decrease the associated morbidity and mortality.

Cancer

Colorectal carcinoma can be considered a disease of the elderly, with an incidence that doubles with each successive decade of life past the age of 50 years.[69] It accounts for approximately two thirds of all GI malignancies in patients over the age of 70 years, and is a leading cause of death in both men and women.[70]

The most common symptom of distal colon and rectal tumors is a change in bowel habits, such as constipation. However, constipation is such a common complaint in the elderly that its significance is often not appreciated by the patient or physician. Other nonspecific complaints, such as weakness, fatigue, vague abdominal discomfort, and changes in mental status, are also frequently attributed to other causes or are disregarded for long periods of time. As a result, the diagnosis is often not made until a complication such as obstruction or perforation occurs.

Diagnosis is often delayed

Diagnostic delays may explain why the depth of invasion in the bowel wall is greater and the need for emergency surgery more frequent in older patients than in younger patients (58% vs 43%).[71] Mortality, which is approximately 4% in the elective setting, triples when emergency surgery becomes necessary.[72] Early detection is essential if the need for emergency surgery and the subsequent mortality is to be reduced. Fecal occult blood screening is not completely satisfactory, as false-negative results have been reported in more than two thirds of patients with Dukes' A and B tumors (Fig. 6).[73] A more aggressive use of colonoscopy has been shown to increase the yield of these early cancers nearly fourfold. Screening with colonoscopy is recommended only for patients felt to be at high risk (eg, patients with previous cancers, previous adenomatous polyps, and ulcerative colitis). Recent data suggest that the protection from death from colorectal cancer provided by sigmoidoscopy lasts for 10 years.[74] If this proves to be true for colonoscopy as well, only infrequent screening would be necessary.[75]

Figure 6

Operative morbidity and mortality as well as long-term survival following the surgical resection of colorectal tumors is not significantly influenced by age. Cancers of the abdominal colon have been resected in patients 80 years of age or older with mortality as low as 2.2% and survival rates comparable to those in younger patients.[76] There has been some reluctance to offer resection for very low rectal cancers to the most elderly patients. Transanal excision, transsacral excision, and fulguration have been used successfully in patients with a short life expectancy or extremely high surgical risk. However, in elderly patients with

Resection

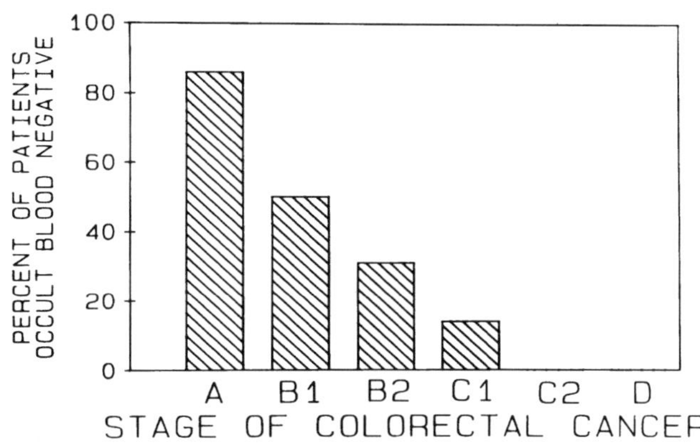

Fig. 6. Graph depicting the percentage of patients with negative stool occult blood tests according to the stage of disease. Note the high percentage of false-negative results in early colorectal tumors. (From Longo, et al.[73] Reprinted with permission.)

little comorbidity, low anterior resection, abdominoperineal resection, and even the newest sphincter-saving coloanal procedures have been performed with mortality similar to that in younger patients.[77] However, the practicality of stomal care must be taken into account in some elderly patients when permanent colostomy is considered.

Obstruction

Volvulus. Colonic volvulus is the third most common cause of large-bowel obstruction in the United States of America, following tumors and diverticulitis. In the majority of cases, the volvulus occurs in the sigmoid colon where an elongated bowel loop twists around a narrow attachment at the base of the mesentery. Volvulus of the cecum is less common, and occurs when the ceum is not firmly attached to the right lateral gutter.

Factors leading to volvulus

In the United States of America, chronic constipation and laxative abuse are thought to be responsible for the development of the elongated, redundant sigmoid loop. Neuropsychiatric disorders also have been observed in a majority of patients with volvulus. Psychotropic medications, chronic debilitation, and protracted immobility concurrently lead to changes in colonic motility, constipation and, eventually, volvulus.

Difficult diagnosis

The clinical presentation of volvulus is difficult to distinguish from that of other causes of large-bowel obstruction or pseudo-obstruction. Abdominal distention, often of great proportions, is the dominant feature. Pain in varying degrees is also common. Previous episodes of similar distention and pain, relieved dramatically by the passage of a large volume of gas and stool, have been reported in well over one third of patients. The general condition of the patient depends on the duration of symptoms and the degree of bowel ischemia present, and can vary from no significant compromise to septic shock. On physical examination distention is constant, but abdominal tenderness and the character of the bowel sounds can vary markedly. Once infarction occurs, signs of peritonitis will prevail.

Sigmoid volvulus without ischemia

In the absence of bowel ischemia, sigmoid volvulus is treated by endoscopic decompression with rigid proctoscopy or colonoscopy. The success rate with either technique varies from 75% to 95%.[78,79] One recent series reported a success rate of 100% in 83 cases, with a mortality of 2.1%.[80] Immediate recurrence is minimized by the insertion of a soft rectal tube at the time of endoscopic decompression. Nonoperative decompression eliminates the need for emergency operation, but is not definitive therapy. Recurrence rates following successful decompression vary from 18% to 35%,[78] but rates as high as 90% have been reported.[81] Decompression should be followed by a thorough bowel preparation and elective sigmoid resection. Operative mortality of ≤5% can be expected.[78]

When endoscopic decompression fails, emergency surgery is mandatory. In this setting there is no consensus about which procedure is best. Simple detorsion is associated with recurrence rates that are too high to justify this approach. Detorsion with resection 1 to 2 weeks after adequate preparation, and detorsion with sigmoidopexy or extraperitonealization of the sigmoid have been advocated. Recently, fixation of the mesentery with synthetic mesh has been proposed.[82]

Sigmoid volvulus with ischemia

Emergency surgery is also indicated when bowel ischemia is suspected. Under these conditions there is general agreement that resection of the compromised bowel with end colostomy and mucous fistula or blind rectal pouch is the procedure of choice.

The most important determinant of outcome with sigmoid volvulus is bowel viability at the time of operation. Mortality jumps from 5% in elective circumstances to 40% in the presence of dead bowel.[78]

Cecal volvulus

Cecal volvulus presents a more difficult problem because the distance of the torsion from the rectum makes it harder to obtain access for nonoperative decompression. Colonoscopic decompression has been effective, although less so than for sigmoid volvulus; thus, emergency operation is required more often. If compromised bowel is present at surgery, right hemicolectomy is indicated. Some investigators have advocated detorsion followed by cecopexy or cecostomy if there is no bowel ischemia. The high recurrence rates of 25% to 35% following cecopexy in some series have led others to advocate right hemicolectomy routinely.[83] Again, mortality is determined by the viability of the bowel and rises from 12% to 15% in the absence of ischemia to nearly 40% in the presence of dead bowel.[84]

Stercoral Ulceration. Stercoral ulcer of the colon, first described by Berry in 1894,[85] is an area of ischemic necrosis of the bowel wall caused by pressure from a hard fecal mass. It is relatively uncommon, found primarily in debilitated elderly patients. Constipation is an almost constant feature. Poor bowel habits and prolonged inactivity are thought to decrease colonic

A problem in debilitated elderly patients

mucus production and lead to the development of rocklike concretions in the rectum and sigmoid. Perforations of stercoral ulcers nearly always occur on the antimesenteric border of the rectosigmoid.

Stercoral ulcers by themselves do not usually produce symptoms and are most often found on routine proctoscopy or colonoscopy. Bleeding occurs in approximately 30% of cases but is rarely significant enough to warrant intervention. Biopsy is necessary to rule out malignancy, but no other local treatment is indicated. Correction of the constipation is the primary goal of therapy.

Stercoral Perforation. This is a disasterous complication with a mortality of 50%.[86,87] Rapid resuscitation and immediate operation are indicated. Resection of the perforated segment and end colostomy have been associated with the lowest mortality (23%),[88] although some advocate exteriorization of the perforation as a loop colostomy, if possible.[86]

Idiopathic large bowel obstruction

Pseudoobstruction. Colonic pseudoobstruction was first recognized by Ogilvie in 1948.[89] Since that time it has been referred to by various names, including Ogilvie's syndrome, idiopathic large-bowel obstruction, colonic ileus, and large intestinal colic. It is seen in association with a variety of disorders, including such illnesses as spinal surgery or injury, cerebrovascular events, neuropsychiatric drug side effects, orthopaedic surgery, diabetic ketoacidosis, myxedema, and rectoperitoneal hematoma. The clinical presentation is fairly constant. Prodigious abdominal distention with little or no pain is the hallmark of this entity. Constipation or obstipation are nearly always present, and nausea and vomiting are nearly always absent. Plain abdominal films will show massive distention of the colon and rectum, with no air-fluid levels (Fig. 7). These findings may be similar to those of sigmoid volvulus or distal mechanical large-bowel obstruction, but patients with these latter disorders usually have a far greater number of symptoms.

Figure 7

The natural history of pseudoobstruction depends on the underlying etiology. When an easily correctable problem (eg, hypokalemia) is responsible for the dilatation, the pseudoobstruction usually resolves once the underlying abnormality is rectified. However, spontaneous resolution can be expected in only one third of cases where no obvious cause can be found.[90]

Medical management

At present, the treatment of pseudoobstruction consists of restriction of oral intake, intravenous hydration, nasogastric decompression, and correction of all predisposing abnormalities. If no cause is found, the diagnosis is uncertain, or correction of the underlying cause fails to relieve the distention, colonoscopy should be performed for diagnosis and decompression. This form of decompression has been successful in nearly 90% of cases, with few complications and a recurrence rate of about 20%.[91]

Surgical management

Surgical management of pseudoobstruction is reserved for patients in whom cecal perforation has occurred or is imminent. A cecal diameter of 9 to 12 cm is said to indicate impeding rupture, but there are no hard data to confirm this, and diameters of up to 25 cm have been reported in patients managed

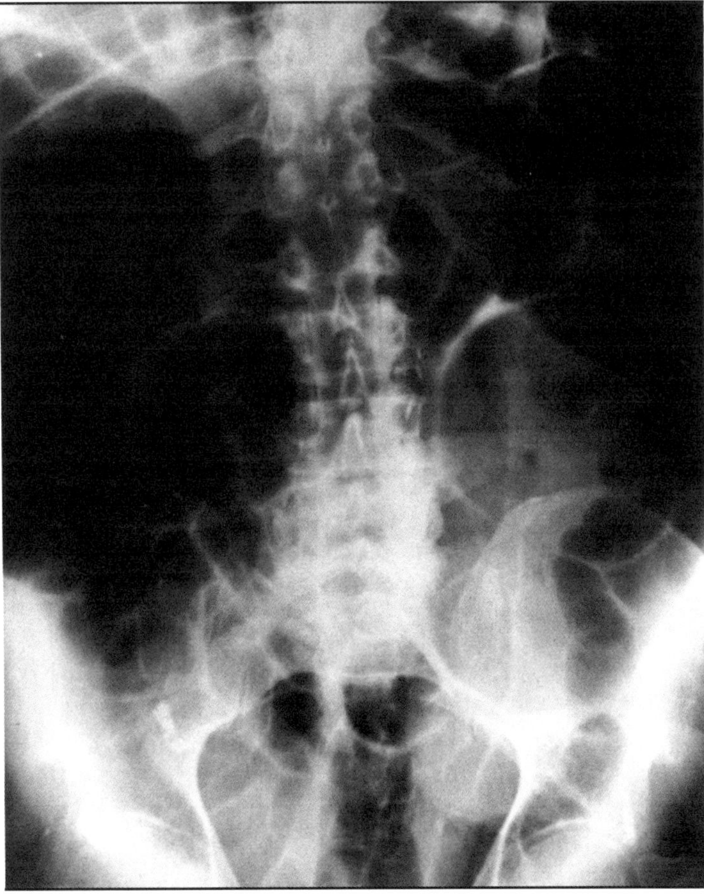

Fig. 7. Abdominal flat plate showing the nonspecific pattern of massive colonic dilation typical of pseudoobstruction.

successfully without operation. Serial films to monitor the progression of the distention are probably more reliable than is a single determination of cecal size.[92] Surgical intervention for pseudoobstruction is often technically challenging and hazardous. Transverse loop colostomy and cecostomy are the two most frequently performed procedures if rupture has not occurred. Resection is indicated when perforation has occurred and the area of ischemia is diffuse. Cecostomy through the perforation is sometimes possible if the ischemic area is small and well demarcated. The operative mortality for all of these procedures is considerable due to the debilitated state of most patients. A valiant attempt at nonoperative decompression should always be made before proceeding with surgery.

Rectal Prolapse

Rectal prolapse has been recognized since 1500 BC, yet the exact etiology and treatment of this uncommon disorder remain controversial.[93] In fact, the term *rectal prolapse* describes a spectrum of disorders that must be differentiated because the treat-ments for each are unique.

Mucosal prolapse

The least functionally significant form of the disorder is mucosal prolapse; it is caused by weakening of the connective tissue between the rectal submucosa and the underlying muscular layers. This allows the mucosa to separate from the bowel wall and prolapse while the muscular wall of the bowel remains in the normal position. Etiologically, it is a separate entity from true prolapse. Treatment is similar to simple hemorrhoidectomy.

Internal prolapse

First-degree prolapse, also called internal rectal prolapse, hidden prolapse, and concealed procidentia, is a prolapse of the full thickness of the wall of the distal sigmoid into the rectal lumen but not through the anal orifice. Some believe that internal prolapse is an early form of true prolapse, although this is not uniformly true. The incidence of progression is estimated to range from 2% to 100%.

True rectal prolapse

True rectal prolapse, also called procidentia, complete prolapse, and overt prolapse, is a circumferential protrusion of the full thickness of the sigmoid into the rectal lumen and through the anal opening. Intussusception of the rectosigmoid into the rectum with a lead point at 6 to 8 cm from the anal verge is generally accepted to be the mechanism of true prolapse.[94] It is thought to be caused by conditions that weaken the pelvic floor, including trauma, iatrogenic injuries, chronic constipation, and congenital predisposition. Intussusception of the rectosigmoid into the rectal lumen occurs when there is increased intra-abdominal pressure, loose rectal attachments, and lax pelvic musculature. Rectal prolapse is frequently accompanied by incontinence. Some believe that incontinence and prolapse are two separate manifestations of pelvic denervation[95] whereas others feel that internal sphincter dysfunction and persistent overdistention of the rectum from constipation predispose to the loss of continence.[96]

The clinical presentation of these disorders depends on the degree of prolapse. A change in bowel habits is usually noted early. Rectal and pelvic pain, a feeling of incomplete evacuation, and tenesmus are common complaints. As the disorder progresses, episodes of fecal soiling and incontinence become more prominent. With true procidentia, the prolapsing segment is usually the presenting complaint. Initially, it may be present only on defecation, but eventually even standing up may cause a sufficient increase in intra-abdominal pressure to result in the appearance of the intussusceptum. The protruding portion is usually edematous and thickened and may bleed or produce mucoid rectal discharge. Patients often learn to reduce the bowel manually with gentle pressure. Incarceration with subsequent gangrene can occur. Rarely, the intussuscepted bowel may rupture and the abdominal contents protrude through the ruptured segment.

Although the association between prolapse and incontinence is not completely defined, it is generally believed that a causal relationship exists. The longer the prolapse is present, the more likely it is that incontinence will develop. If continence has not already been disturbed, early repair is strongly advised. Numerous surgical procedures have been used with varying success. However, most studies have involved small numbers of patients so no one procedure has emerged as best. These operations are performed via an abdominal or perineal approach.

Transabdominal surgery

The Abdominal Approach. In general, transabdominal repairs of rectal prolapse have been very successful. However, they usually require general anesthesia and expose patients to all of the potential complications of laparotomy. The most well-known transabdominal procedure is the pelvic sling repair, popularized by Ripstein.[97] In this operation, the rectum is mobilized and the intussusception is reduced. The rectum is then fixed to the sacrum using a circumferential sling made of foreign material. In the original description, a 360° Teflon wrap was used. Both the material and the degrees of wrap have changed over the years.[98] Teflon, which was thought to be too inert, was replaced with Marlex, which was too reactive. Most recently, Gortex has been used with good results. The 360° wraps, which were felt to lead to fecal impaction, have been replaced with wraps that leave a portion of the wall unincorporated, to allow for some distention. These sling procedures have been associated with low recurrence (0% to 4%) and operative mortality (2%). However, complications (eg, fecal impaction, bleeding, stricture, pelvic abscess, impotence) occur in 17% of cases and can be serious.[99]

Theoretically, posterior rectopexy (Wells procedure), can obviate some of these complications.[100] In this operation, the rectum is fixed to the sacrum posteriorly by insertion of a reactive material, initially an Ivalon sponge, between the rectum and the sacrum. The inflammatory reaction generated by the foreign body causes scarring and fibrosis. By not encircling the rectum, the problems of fecal impaction and stricture could be avoided. Although the incidence of these complications is decreased by this procedure, pelvic sepsis from the foreign material may occur, and recurrence rates are as high as 10%.[101]

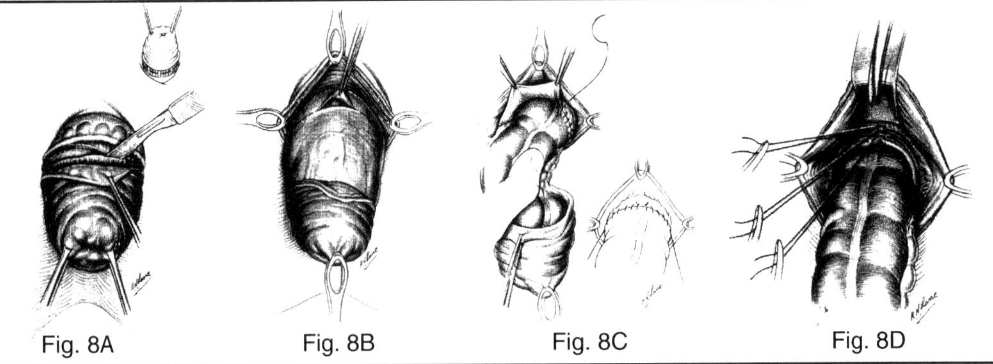

Fig. 8. Rectosigmoidectomy. **(A)** A circumferential full-thickness incision is made in the prolapsed bowel 3 cm from the dentate line. **(B)** The pouch of Douglas is identified on the anterior aspect of the bowel and is opened. **(C)** The sigmoid is pulled down through the opening and the anterior cut edge of the peritoneum is sutured to the serosa of the bowel. **(D)** The puborectalis is sutured together anterior to the bowel. (From Galligher J, in Galligher J [ed]. *Surgery of the Anus, Rectum and Colon*, ed 5, London, Balliére Tindall, 1984, pp 246-284. Reprinted with permission.)

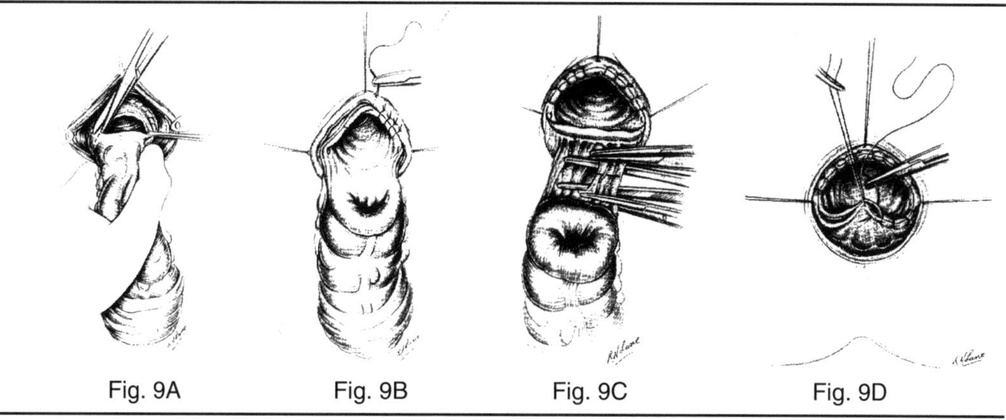

Fig. 9. Rectosigmoidectomy. **(A)** The colon is incised anteriorly approximately 2 cm distal to the peritoneal suture line. **(B)** Stay sutures are placed anteriorly and laterally and the full thickness of the rectal stump is sutured to the full-thickness cut edge of the sigmoid. **(C)** The posterior wall of the sigmoid is divided and the mesorectum is divided and ligated. **(D)** The remaining posterior of the sigmoid is sutured to the posterior rectal stump. (From Galligher J, in Galligher J [ed]. *Surgery of the Anus, Rectum and Colon*, ed 5, London, Balliére Tindall, 1984, pp 246-284. Reprinted with permission).

Posterior rectopexy

Simple posterior rectopexy or direct fixation of the rectum to the sacrum with nonabsorbable suture material has gained fairly wide acceptance. Several series have reported no recurrence and 0% mortality with this approach, but only 72% to 80% of patients in these series had subjectively good or excellent results.[102] Resection in combination with posterior rectopexy has been advocated, but complication rates as high as 30% have been reported, related mostly to the anastomosis. Simple resection has been advocated as well, but this is associated with recurrence rates approaching 10%, and high complication rates.[103]

Perineal approach to avoid laparotomy

The Perineal Approach. The perineal approach to rectal prolapse is advantageous because it avoids the potential complications associated with laparotomy and usually is performed under regional rather than general anesthesia. The simplest of the perineal procedures involves encircling the anus with a silver wire, as described initially by Thiersch. This prevents the bowel from exiting the anal orifice but does nothing to actually correct the intussusception. Therefore, it is viewed as a palliative procedure, which is rarely necessary, unless the patient has a truly prohibitive operative risk.

Figures 8 and 9

The best perineal procedure is the perineal rectosigmoidectomy popularized by Altemeier (Figs. 8 and 9).[104] In this operation, an incision is made in the prolapsing segment several centimeters proximal to the dentate line. The full thickness of the bowel wall is incised around the full circumference until the underlying rectosigmoid and mesocolon are visualized. The pouch of Douglas on the anterior surface of the rectosigmoid is then opened, and the sigmoid is pulled down firmly, with any slack removed. The pouch is reconstructed by suturing the anterior peritoneal edge to the surface of the sigmoid as high as possible. The levator on either side can then be palpated and approximated in the midline with several stitches. Following this, the mesocolon is divided, as is the prolapsed segment of bowel, and continuity is restored by suturing the transected edge to the anal cuff. Transient incontinence is common postoperatively, but usually resolves within 1 to 2 months. In the hands of advocates, recurrence rates for this procedure are low,[105] although this has not been the experience in general. Complication rates are low as well.[105] Although these procedures have not gained widespread acceptance, they are most useful in elderly patients in whom laparotomy presents an inordinate risk. They can be performed safely, with minimal postoperative impairment and rapid recovery.

References

1. Nelsen JB, Castell DO, in Hazard WR, et al (eds). *Principles of Geriatric Medicine and Gerontology*, ed 2, New York, McGraw Hill, 1990, pp 593-608.
2. Robertson GS, et al. *Digestion* 1988;40:244-246.
3. Scott HW Jr, et al. *South Med J* 1985;78:1309-1311.
4. Stipa S, et al. *Surg Gynecol Obstet* 1990;170:212-216.
5. Castell DO. *Gastoenterol Clin North Am* 1990;19:235.
6. Attwood SEA, et al. *Br J Surg* 1992;79:1050-1053.
7. Mercer CD, Hill LD. *Thorac Cardiovasc Surg* 1986;91:371-378.
8. Vallan G, et al. *Eur J Surg* 1992;158:357-360.
9. Sugimachi K, et al. *Br J Surg* 1985;72:28-31.
10. Muehrcke DD, et al. *Thorax* 1989;44:141-145.
11. Keeling P, et al. *Ann Royal Coll Surg Engl* 1988;70:34-37.
12. Willianson RCN. *Ann Royal Coll Surg Engl* 1985;67:344-348.
13. Nishi M, et al. *Ann Surg* 1988;207:148-154.
14. Perez-Perez GI, et al. *Ann Intern Med* 1988;109:11-17.
15. Graham DY, et al. *J Infect Dis* 1988;157:777-780.
16. Bird T, et al. *Gerontology* 1977;23:309-315.
17. Permutt RP, Cello JP. *Dig Dis Sci* 1982;27:1-6.
18. *World Health Organization Statistics Annual 1988*. Geneva, World Health Organization 1988.
19. Galinsky NH. *Gastroenterol Clin North Am* 1990;19:255-272.
20. Watson RJ, et al. *Age Aging* 1985;14:225-229.
21. Scapa E, et al. *J Clin Gastroenterol* 1989;11:502-506.
22. Griffin MR, et al. *Ann Intern Med* 1991;14:257-263.
23. Collier DSJ, Pain JA. *Gut* 1985;26:359-363.
24. Somerville K, et al. *Lancet* 1986;1:462-466.
25. Clinch D, Banerjee AK. *Age Aging* 1985;13:120-123.
26. Kaplan MS, et al. *Arch Surg* 1972;104:667-671.
27. Walt R, et al. *Lancet* 1986;1:489-492.
28. Coleman JA, Denham MJ. *Age Aging* 1980;9:251-257.
29. Boey T, et al. *Ann Surg* 1982;196:338-344.
30. Rosenthal RA, et al, in Katlic MR (ed). *Geriatric Surgery*, Baltimore, Md, Urban & Schwarzenberg, Inc, 1990, pp 459-512.
31. Stanfford CE, et al. *Calif Med* 1956;84:92-94.
32. Amberg JR, Zboralske FF. *Am J Roentgenol* 1966;96:393-399.
33. Jordan PH Jr, in Scott WH, Sawyers JL (eds). *Surgery of the Stomach, Duodenum and Small Intestines*, Boston, Mass, Blackwell Scientific Publications, 1987, pp 395-426.
34. Sun DCH, Stempien SJ. *Gastroenterology* 1971;61:576-584.
35. Adkins RB, et al. *Ann Surg* 1985;201:741-751.
36. Jensen HE, et al. *Scand J Gastroenterol* 1972;7:535-540.
37. Green LK, Graham DY. *Gastroenterol Clin North Am* 1990;19:273-292.
38. Coluccia C, et al. *Int Surg* 1987;72:4-10.
39. Bandoh T, et al. *Surgery* 1991;109:136-142.
40. Edelman DS, et al. *Am Surg* 1987;53:170-173.
41. Holt P. *Gastroenterol Clin North Am* 1990;19:345-360.
42. Zadeh BJ, et al. *Am Surg* 1985;51:470-473.
43. Mucha P Jr. *Surg Clin North Am* 1987;67:597-620.
44. Green WW. *Am J Surg* 1969;118:541-545.
45. Ishitani MB, Jones RS, in Scott HW, Sawyers JL (eds). *Surgery of the Stomach, Duodenum and Small Intestines*, Boston, Mass, Blackwell Scientific Publications, 1987, pp 877-900.
46. Deysine M, et al. *Am J Surg* 1987;153:387-391.
47. Lewis DC, et al. *J Royal Coll Surg Edinburgh* 1989;32:101-103.

48. Temple TF, Miller RE. *J Natl Med Assoc* 1980;72:513-515.
49. Awrich AE, et al. *Surg Gynecol Obstet* 1980;151:9-14.
50. Dial P, Cohn I, in Scott HW, Sawyers JL (eds). *Surgery of the Stomach, Duodenum and Small Intestines*, Boston, Mass, Blackwell Scientific Publications, 1987, pp 937-952.
51. Swan RW, Fowler WC Jr. *Surg Gynecol Obstet* 1976;142:325-329.
52. Swift RI, et al. *J Royal Coll Surg Edinburgh* 1989;34:267-269.
53. Stalnickowicz R, et al. *J Clin Gastroenterol* 1989;11:411-415.
54. Watts JM, et al. *Gut* 1966;7:16-20.
55. Zimmerman J, et al. *J Clin Gastroenterol* 1985;7:492-496.
56. Grimm IS, Friedman LS. *Gastroenterol Clin North Am* 1990;18:361-390.
57. Jones HW, Hoare AM. *Age Aging* 1988;17:410-414.
58. Frabicius PJ, et al. *Gut* 1985;26:461-465.
59. Boley SJ, et al. *Surg Gynecol Obstet* 1981;153:561-566.
60. Boley SJ, et al. *Surgery* 1972;82:848-854.
61. Boley SJ, Brandt LJ. *Dig Dis Sci* 1986;31(supplement):26S-42S.
62. Cheskin LJ, et al. *Gastroenterol Clin North Am* 1990;19:391-404.
63. Boley SJ, et al. *Clin Gastroenterol* 1981;10:65-91.
64. Reinus JF, et al. *Gastroenterol Clin North Am* 1990;19:319-344.
65. Boyd BJ, et al. *Ann Surg* 1981;192:743-746.
66. Finley IG, Carter CC. *Dis Colon Rectum* 1987;30:920-933.
67. Lau WY, et al. *Surg Gynecol Obstet* 1985;161:157-160.
68. Hall A, Wright T. *Am Surg* 1976;42:147-150.
69. Weilaw B. *Clin Geriatr Med* 1987;3:625-635.
70. Wallach CB, Kurtz RC. *Gastroenterol Clin North Am* 1990;19:419-432.
71. Waldon RD, et al. *Br J Surg* 1986;73:314-317.
72. Webbes TH. *Age Aging* 1985;14:321-323.
73. Longo WE, et al. *Ann Surg* 1988;207:174-179.
74. Selby JV, et al. *N Engl J Med* 1992;326:653-657.
75. Ransohoff DF, Lang CA. *JAMA* 1993;269:1278-1281.
76. Habler KE. *Am Surg* 1986;203:129-131.
77. Huguet C, et al. *World J Surg* 1990;14:619-622.
78. Ballantyne UH. *Dis Colon Rectum* 1982;25:795-798.
79. Mangiante EL, et al. *Am Surg* 1989;55:41-44.
80. Arigbabu AO, et al. *Dis Colon Rectum* 1985;28:795-798.
81. Hines RJ, et al. *Surg Gynecol Obstet* 1967;124:567-570.
82. Hellman AA, Cramer WO. *Surg Gynecol Obstet* 1988;167:249-250.
83. Parhlman L, et al. *Acta Chir Scand* 1989;155:53-56.
84. Ballantyne GH, et al. *Ann Surg* 1985;202:83-92.
85. Berry J. *Br Med J* 1984;297:301-305.
86. Maull KI, et al. *Am Surg* 1982;48:20-24.
87. Gekas D, Shuster MN. *Gastroenterology* 1981;80:1054-1058.
88. Guyton DP, et al. *Am Surg* 1985;51:520-522.
89. Ogilvie H. *Br J Med* 1948;2:671-673.
90. Bullock PR, Thomas WE. *Ann Royal Coll Surg Engl* 1984;66:327-329.
91. Nano D, et al. *Am J Gastroenterol* 1987;82:142-148.
92. Baker DA, et al. *JAMA* 1979;241:263-264.
93. Lawry AL, Goldberg SM. *Surg Clin North Am* 1987;16:47-70.
94. Broden B, Snellman B. *Dis Colon Rectum* 1968;11:330-349.
95. Snook SJ, et al. *Gut* 1985;26:470-476.
96. Cherry DA, Rothenberger DA. *Surg Clin North Am* 1988;68:1217-1230.
97. Ripstein CB. *Dis Colon Rectum* 1965;8:34-48.
98. Roberts PL, et al. *Arch Surg* 1988;123:554-557.
99. Holstrom B, et al. *Dis Colon Rectum* 1986;29:845-848.
100. Atkinson KG, Taylor DC. *Dis Colon Rectum* 1984;27:96-98.
101. Lake SA, et al. *Dis Colon Rectum* 1989;27:589-590.
102. Carter AE. *Br J Surg* 1983;70:522-523.
103. Graham W, et al. *Ann Royal Coll Surg Engl* 1984;66:87-89.
104. Altemeier WA, Culbertson WR. *Surgery* 1965;58:758-764.
105. Prasad ML, et al. *Dis Colon Rectum* 1986;29:547-552.
106. Cutler CW. *Surg Gynecol Obstet* 1958;107:23-30.

III Hepatobiliary and Pancreatic Disease in the Elderly

Joel J. Roslyn, MD
Kim U. Kahng, MD

BRIEF CONTENTS

INTRODUCTION

Hepatobiliary procedures account for approximately 20% of all abdominal operations performed in people over the age of 65 years in the United States of America.[1] This underscores the need for a clear understanding of the diseases affecting the liver, gallbladder, biliary tract, and pancreas in the geriatric population. This issue assumes greater importance when we recognize that more emergency biliary tract procedures are performed in the elderly than in younger patients.[2,3] In addition, the incidence of significant complications from cholelithiasis is increased among the elderly.[4-6]

Advances in radiologic, endoscopic and, most recently, laparoscopic technologies, in combination with our expanding knowledge and understanding of the systemic manifestations of hyperbilirubinemia, have provided the background and impetus for new and innovative approaches to the management of elderly patients with hepatobiliary and pancreatic disorders.

Formulation of a management strategy for the elderly

The consideration of issues unique to geriatric surgery is essential prior to and during the formulation of a management strategy for the elderly patient with hepatobiliary or pancreatic disease. Several studies have suggested that the most significant determinant of mortality in elderly patients undergoing cholecystectomy is the presence of cardiovascular or cerebrovascular disease.[7,8] The relationship between hyperbilirubinemia and renal dysfunction[9] may be critical in elderly patients, many of whom already have some element of renal insufficiency. Many biliary disorders are manifested or complicated by the presence of cholangitis. The development of this severe variant of biliary sepsis may be life-threatening in elderly patients, who are more susceptible to the consequences of systemic hypoperfusion.

Perhaps the most challenging issues confronting today's physicians caring for elderly patients with hepatobiliary or pancreatic disorders relate to the ethical and philosophical considerations associated with malignancies arising in these organs. Given the grave prognosis inherent with many of these lesions, it is incumbent upon the surgeon to measure the relative merits of radical resection and palliation. In addition to the obvious medical issues, careful consideration must be given to such social issues as quality of life, the patient's ability to recognize and deal emotionally with the prognosis of the underlying malady, provision of long-term care and in what setting, and rehabilitative potential.

PHYSIOLOGIC CHANGES

Aging is associated with specific alterations in the morphologic and physiologic function of the liver, gallbladder, and pancreas. But of possibly greater importance are the systemic changes that occur with aging, specifically the well-documented changes in host defense mechanisms that may predispose to infection and sepsis. These changes include altered cell-mediated function, humoral T-cell response, and a nonspecific alteration in the integrity of the skin and mucus membranes, which may facilitate susceptibility to postoperative wound infection.

LIVER DISEASE

Hepatic function changes little

The liver undergoes significant morphologic changes with aging, including a reduction in absolute and relative size[10] and molding to conform to adjacent organs.[11] In addition, hepatic blood flow diminishes by a small but measurable amount each year, such that total liver blood flow is 40% lower in patients over the age of 60 years than in patients under the age of 25 years.[12] Other changes in liver architecture include a reduction in hepatocytes and bile duct proliferation.[13] Yet, the clinical significance of these changes remains unclear. In fact, considerable evidence suggests that hepatic function remains normal during aging, as manifested by normal total bilirubin, alkaline phosphatase, and aspartate aminotransferase levels,[14] normal biliary excretion of sodium sulfobromophthalein,[15] and normal metabolism of most drugs.[16]

Cholesterol saturation of bile

Clinical data have documented an increased incidence of cholesterol gallstones associated with aging in both men and women.[17] As a person ages, the activities of specific hepatic enzymes critical to cholesterol biosynthesis are altered, with a decrease in 7-α-hydroxylase and an increase in 3-hydroxy-3-methylglutaryl coenzyme A (HMG-CoA) reductase.[18] The net effect of these changes is an increase in the degree of cholesterol saturation of bile. The factors responsible for this change are unclear, although alterations in the ratios of androgen to estrogen have been the focus of recent investigations.

Metastatic Cancer

Malignant tumors of the liver are seen considerably more frequently in elderly patients than are benign tumors; thus, the finding of a filling defect on ultrasonography or computed tomography (CT) is reason for grave concern. The overwhelming majority of metastatic lesions in the liver arise from a primary gastrointestinal site; colorectal carcinomas are most common. The surgical management of colorectal metastases to the liver has assumed increasing importance in recent years as a result of a number of related advances. These include earlier diagnosis facilitated by routine surveillance, improved preoperative and intraoperative assessment, and new insights into segmental resections and liver-conserving procedures. In addition, data from various centers throughout the world suggest that hepatic resection of colorectal metastases improves the survival of patients with isolated hepatic disease.[19-21]

Factors influencing disease-free interval and survival

While a number of factors have been carefully analyzed for impact on survival, the effect of age has not been well defined. Yet, age itself is not as important to this decision-making process as is a patient's overall medical and mental state and factors related to the tumor. The presence of portal/celiac nodes, length of tumor-free margin of resection, distribution and number of metastases, and stage of the primary cancer have been shown to influence disease-free interval and survival. Each of these factors should be weighed carefully when considering hepatic resection in this clinical setting. Obstruction of the major bile ducts can occur in the presence of metastatic cancer and may be due to tumor debris or extrinsic compression.[22] Intubation of the biliary tract usually provides good palliation for affected patients and generally can be achieved without significant morbidity or mortality.

Primary Malignancy

The recent identification of specific etiologic factors in the development of hepatoma, coupled with the worldwide frequency with which this tumor occurs, has been responsible for intense investigative and clinical interest. Hepatoma, the most common of all primary liver tumors, ranks only 22nd among cancers treated in the United States of America.[23] Hepatocellular carcinoma is more common in men than in women, and its incidence increases with age. However, there appears to be a leveling off of this rise in the elderly population.

Diagnosis of hepatocellular carcinoma

Ultrasonography and CT have varying sensitivities in diagnosing hepatocellular carcinoma.[23-25] Ultrasound or CT-guided biopsy can be performed percutaneously, but the most sensitive test for diagnosing hepatoma is visceral angiography.[26] Caution should be exercised primarily because of the potential vascular and nephrologic sequelae. We typically reserve angiography for the older patient with a suspicious lesion in whom hepatic resection would be considered.

Resection

Cholangiocarcinomas account for approximately 15% of primary hepatic tumors. These lesions typically spread in a diffuse manner throughout the liver, and the opportunity for resection is limited. This is in contrast to extrahepatic bile duct tumors, for which there is increasing enthusiasm for radical resection.

Hepatic resection for malignant disease is being performed with increasing frequency throughout the world. In many centers the perioperative mortality is less than 10%.[27-29] The role of age as a determinant of outcome following major hepatic resection remains unclear. In a retrospective review, Ezaki et al[30] showed that hepatic resection can be performed safely in the elderly, and that the factors that determine outcome are linked more to preoperative liver function and histology than to age.

Benign Tumors and Cysts

The majority of benign lesions of the liver are hepatic adenomas, focal nodular hyperplasias, hemangiomas, and solitary cysts. Hepatic adenomas and focal nodular lesions tend to be found in women of childbearing age and generally are not associated with the elderly. Although hemangiomas have been identified among elderly patients, they are noted with much greater frequency among patients in the third, fourth, and fifth decades of life.

Hemangiomas and solitary cysts

Asymptomatic lesions that are discovered in elderly patients should be managed similarly to those found in younger patients. Solitary cysts tend to be congenital, but their pattern of slow growth makes their presentation in later life not at all uncommon. Most of these lesions are located in the right lobe and typically contain clear fluid. When symptoms are present, they are generally related to extrinsic compression on the stomach, resulting in some element of early satiety. Such patients receive

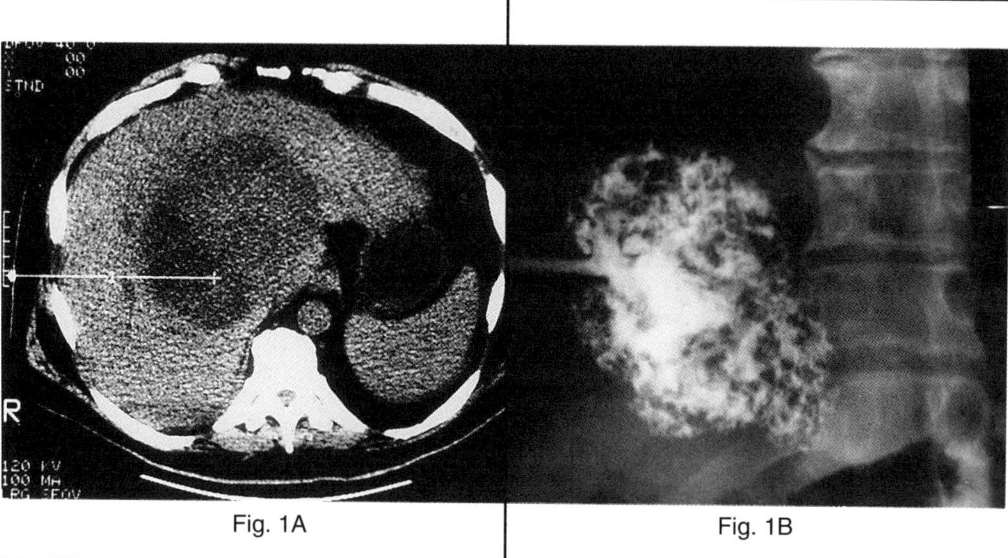

Fig.1. (A) Computed tomogram of a 76-year-old man who presented with low-grade fever, malaise, and weight loss. During evaluation his fever spiked and a central hepatic abscess was discovered. This scan shows the placement of a percutaneous drain. Ultimately, the focus was identified as diverticulitis. (B) Tubogram demonstrating radiographically the size of the abscess cavity. This required no further intervention and resolved over the course of several weeks. The patient subsequently underwent sigmoid colectomy and has had no further problems.

enormous benefit from cyst decompression. Simple unroofing of these cysts (with biopsy to exclude cystadenocarcinoma) or Roux-en-Y cystojejunostomy (if the cyst contains bile) can be accomplished with minimal morbidity and may provide considerable relief.

Abscess

At one time the most common cause of liver abscess was appendicitis; now it is biliary tract disease.[31] Therefore, it is not surprising that hepatic abscess is emerging as an important problem in the elderly. Many elderly patients will have indolent presentations with no antecedent infection demonstrated. Diagnosis can be confirmed by ultrasonography or CT. Surgical drainage of hepatic abscesses has long been the gold standard for treatment, but enthusiasm has been growing for percutaneous drainage as a primary modality (Fig. 1).[32,33] Long-term follow-up data with percutaneous drainage is essential to understanding its role in the management of these patients. This modality is particularly appealing in the elderly, but standard surgical principles for management should be followed.

Figure 1

GALLBLADDER DISEASE

The effects of aging on gallbladder and pancreatic function have not been well defined. Attention has been focused on the relationship of aging to the propensity to form gallstones. The alterations in hepatic metabolism that may contribute to this phenomenon have already been discussed. Ultrasonographic

Regulatory peptides and gallstone formation

studies indicate that gallbladder sensitivity to cholecystokinin (CCK), the primary hormonal stimulus for gallbladder contraction, decreases with age,[34] and serum concentrations of pancreatic polypeptide increase with age.[35] Experimental data suggest that pancreatic polypeptide effects postcontractile gallbladder filling.[36] Further studies are needed to clarify the effects of these and other peptides on hepatobiliary and pancreatic function in the elderly.

Cholelithiasis

Gallstone disease is the most common indication for abdominal surgery among the elderly.[37] This reflects the incidence of cholelithiasis in this age group.

Table 1

Incidence. Numerous studies have demonstrated a linear increase in the prevalence of gallstones with advancing age (Table 1).[37-39] The actual frequency with which gallstones are found in any country or among any ethnic group varies considerably and depends upon a variety of factors. In the United States of America, the incidence of gallstones in Caucasian women increases from 5% at 20 years of age to 12% at 40 years of age, and up to 25% by 60 years of age. Similar trends have been noted in men, although the absolute prevalence remains less than that among women of any given age.

Natural History. Controversy exists regarding the optimal management of elderly patients with asymptomatic gallstones. Considerable evidence suggests that gallstone disease in the elderly may be more virulent than in a younger population. Clinical experience indicates a 50% incidence of choledocholithiasis in patients with gallstones who are over the age of 65 years but less than a 12% incidence of choledocholithiasis in younger patients with gallstones.[40,41] In addition, elderly patients are at an increased risk of developing emphysematous cholecystitis,[42] gallbladder perforation,[43] and septic complications of cholecystitis.[44] This is of particular concern when one considers that recent innovations in laparoscopic surgery, in combination with other extraneous factors, have resulted in some noticeable trends in the management of patients with gallstone disease. A recent study from Israel has demonstrated that patients undergoing cholecystectomy for acute cholecystitis

Table 1. Incidence of Gallbladder Disease by Age

Patient Age (yr)	Patients With Stones	
	Women	Men
10–39	5%	1%
40–49	12%	4%
50–59	16%	6%
60–69	25%	10%
70–79	29%	15%
80–89	31%	18%
≥90	35%	24%

are more likely to be older, diabetic men in whom there is a greater incidence of choledocholithiasis, acalculous cholecystitis, and gangrene, and in whom emergent or urgent surgery will be required.[45] We believe that the increased incidence of problems in the elderly can be attributed to a reluctance on the part of many physicians and surgeons to recommend early elective surgery in older patients with cholelithiasis.

Delay in operative management and complications

The issue of asymptomatic versus symptomatic stone treatment is even more obscure in the geriatric population than it is in younger patients. What constitutes an asymptomatic patient, and how does one define this nebulous entity in an elderly patient who may have numerous other complaints or be mentally incapable of specifying complaints? In an elderly patient with a variety of nonspecific functional or physiologic complaints it may be difficult for the clinician to define an exact cause-and-effect relationship. Clinical experience suggests that many patients will have dyspepsia, vague epigastric discomfort, or even mildly increased flatulence as the primary manifestation of their gallstones. A recent study has suggested that many of these patients will benefit significantly from cholecystectomy.[46]

An interesting and provocative analysis by Ransohoff and Gracie[47] addresses the question of whether patients with an episode of biliary colic require immediate cholecystectomy or only observation until their symptoms recur or a complication develops. Based on a series of assumptions and a computer model, these authors attempted to quantitate the risks of expectant management and operative intervention in patients with symptomatic gallstones. They concluded that "Some patients and physicians may decide that the risk of symptomatic gallstones is low enough that a policy of expectant management may be acceptable." Although this study did not look specifically at elderly patients, it nonetheless will be cited as a reason to support nonoperative therapy for older patients with symptomatic gallstone disease. This type of reasoning may be responsible for the delay in appropriate intervention that is thought to account for the increased incidence of serious complications of gallstones in the elderly.

Expectant vs operative management

Ultimately, the decision to recommend open or laparoscopic cholecystectomy must be based on a number of individual, patient-specific factors. Although we do not routinely advocate prophylactic cholecystectomy in an elderly patient with truly asymptomatic gallstones, we do consider removal of the gallbladder to be appropriate in certain settings. A number of studies have indicated the safety of incidental cholecystectomy in patients undergoing major abdominal surgery.[48,49] The value of this approach is underscored by the recognition that postoperative cholecystitis can be a lethal complication of an otherwise routine procedure.[50] For patients with symptomatic gallstone disease, the primary physician and surgeon need to weigh the potential risks and benefits of an elective procedure based on current data and patient profile. The desire to be conservative must be tempered by the realization that emergent cholecystectomy in the elderly is associated with a significant increase in perioperative mortality.

Open vs laparoscopic surgery

Table 2. Open Cholecystectomy: Effect of Age on Outcome

	Age <65 Yr	Age >65 Yr
Patients (no.)	30,059	12,415
Percentage of Group	70.8%	29.2%
Morbidity	10.2%	25.7%*
Deaths (no.)	9	62
Mortality	0.03%	0.5%*
Hospital stay (d)	4.7	7.3
Charges ($)	5,980	9,728

*P <0.0001 vs age <65 yr.
From Roslyn and Binns.[51]

Treatment. The problem of how to optimize treatment of the elderly with gallstone disease is compounded by the management options for patients with recurrent biliary colic. The introduction and development of new and innovative approaches to gallstone therapy has revolutionized our thinking. In addition to open cholecystectomy, available options include laparoscopic removal of the gallbladder, medical dissolution with pharmaco-logic agents, percutaneous transhepatic cholecystolitholysis (contact dissolution), and biliary lithotripsy.

Open cholecystectomy

Open cholecystectomy continues to be a safe and effective means of dealing with gallstones, and is performed in most hospitals throughout the world. Outcome is most closely linked to age and the presence of comorbid factors. A contemporary computer analysis assessed the effect of age on outcome among 42,474 patients undergoing cholecystectomy during a 1-year period.[51] There were 12,415 patients over the age of 65 years, comprising 29.2% of the total group. Morbidity was 25.7% and mortality was 0.5% (Table 2). Although these figures were significantly greater than those for patients under the age of 65 years, most authorities would consider them very acceptable for patients in this age group undergoing any type of surgery. The dramatic improvement in outcome documented in this recent study compared with a large 1975 longitudinal study[52] reflects the significant advances in perioperative care we have witnessed during the past decade. Similar data have been reported from Europe.[53] Comorbid factors associated with an adverse outcome in these recent studies included the presence of congestive heart failure, a recent myocardial infarction, atrial fibrillation, and cirrhosis. These findings are consistent with those of previous reports, which indicate that outcome following cholecystectomy is determined more by overall medical status than by extent of gallbladder disease.[7,8]

Table 2

Laparoscopic cholecystectomy

In 1988 the treatment of cholelithiasis was revolutionized by the introduction of laparoscopic cholecystectomy.[54] Since then, laparoscopic removal of the gallbladder has become the preferred method of treatment for patients with symptomatic gallstones.[55-60] There are several theoretical advantages to this procedure compared with conventional surgery: reduced hospital stay, easier postoperative recovery, reduced patient discomfort, and a high degree of patient acceptance. Nonetheless, credentialling issues and the safety of this procedure in terms of bile duct injury continue to be subjects of considerable controversy.[61-64] The applicability of laparoscopic cholecystectomy in the elderly has not been addressed specifically, and only now are data emerging regarding the ventilatory effects of carbon dioxide insufflation and laparoscopic cholecystectomy. Unfortunately, initial reports have been contradictory, and the issue remains unclear.[65,66] Greater experience needs to be reported with laparoscopic surgery in the elderly before its role in the management of gallstone disease can be assessed fully.

Pharmacologic dissolution of stones

Dissolution of existing gallstones with pharmacologic agents and the subsequent avoidance of surgery has long been a goal of many investigators and clinicians. This technique would be particularly attractive for elderly patients who may be viewed as poor operative risks by virtue of their comorbid illnesses and reduced recuperative abilities. The recognition that hepatic secretion of cholesterol-saturated bile is a prerequisite for stone formation has prompted numerous attempts at gallstone dissolution by a reduction of bile lithogenicity. Several agents are commercially available and are varyingly efficacious in the dissolution of cholesterol gallstones. Chenodeoxycholic acid (CDCA) has been studied extensively through data collected as part of the National Cooperative Gallstone Study.[67] However, results from over 900 patients have demonstrated a partial response in approximately 28% of cases and complete stone disappearance in less than 15% of additional cases. These disappointing findings are compounded by a 5-year 50% recurrence rate, significant side effects, and the cost of 1 to 2 years of therapy and follow-up.

Ursodeoxycholic acid (UDCA) has been hailed as better, safer, and more effective for gallstone dissolution than is CDCA, particularly in the elderly.[68] However, current estimates suggest that no more than 10% of patients with gallstones in the United States of America would be suitable candidates for either of these agents. What role, if any, should these agents play in the management of elderly patients with gallstones? This question remains largely unanswered, although it is becoming increasingly apparent that their utility as a primary modality is limited.

Methyl-tert-butyl ether (MTBE), an aliphatic ether, is a potent solvent of cholesterol. Although MTBE can be toxic to certain tissues, it is well tolerated when instilled in the gallbladder for short periods of time, and can result in effective cholesterol gallstone dissolution in carefully selected patients with cholesterol stones.[69]

Direct contact dissolution (percutaneous transhepatic cholecystolitholysis) is a relatively new procedure that is based on the ability to place a catheter through the liver into the gallbladder percutaneously, using techniques long employed by interventional radiologists. Complications with this procedure are largely technical and related to catheter placement. As with any procedure that leaves the gallbladder intact, gallstone recurrence is a major drawback, with 50% recurrence predicted at 5 years. No data specifically address the role of this modality in the geriatric population.

Electroshock wave lithotripsy

Electroshock wave lithotripsy (ESWL) was introduced several years ago, and there was great anticipation that this technology would become the universal treatment for patients with symptomatic gallstone disease.[70] Potential advantages include shortened hospital stay, avoidance of surgical intervention and associated complications, and a high rate of acceptance by patients. This noninvasive procedure was particularly attractive for the treatment of elderly patients, as gallstone fragmentation and disappearance presumably could be achieved in most patients over a relatively short period of time. The efficacy of this technique is linked to specific characteristics, including number and size of stones, type of stone and amount of calcium present, status of gallbladder on oral cholecystography, and presence or absence of complications, such as cholecystitis.[71] Unfortunately, data suggest that, using currently accepted inclusion criteria, only 20% of patients would be suitable candidates for this modality.[72] Significant questions remain regarding the cost-effectiveness of the procedure, and a recently completed computer analysis has suggested that ESWL would be cost-effective in only a very small, carefully selected segment of the population with symptomatic gallstone disease.[73]

Acute Cholecystitis

The incidence of cholecystitis has increased significantly over the last several decades in many groups of patients, including those over the age of 70 years. Currently, acute cholecystitis is one of the more common indications for the emergency admission of elderly patients to a surgical service. Recent data suggest that the rate of cholecystitis has increased significantly. However, it is unclear whether this finding represents a true change in the disease process or reflects an evolving health care system that has been influenced by changes in reimbursement strategies and other external influences.[74]

Clinical Presentation. Although the classical manifestations of acute cholecystitis (eg, persistent right upper quadrant pain, fever, leukocytosis) may be present in the elderly, the clinical course is often atypical. Therefore, it is essential that clinicians have a high index of suspicion and consider this diagnosis in elderly patients presenting with abdominal pain or other signs of sepsis. Abdominal pain continues to be the predominant complaint in more than 70% of elderly patients with documented acute cholecystitis.[75] Fever, nausea, and emesis are frequent complaints as well, and may be the only signs of an intra-abdominal process. A palpable mass is noted in approximately 20% of these patients. Even in the absence of choledocholithiasis, jaundice may be a significant finding. Perhaps most distressing is a recent report that 12% of 131 patients over the age of 70 years who presented with acute cholelithiasis were in septic shock at the time of admission.[75] Although the mechanism by which acute cholecystitis occurs is not clear, alterations in mental status have been noted in elderly patients with this disorder.[76] Deterioration in intellectual function may be the primary manifestation of

Pain and signs of sepsis dictate a high index of suspicion

hepatobiliary disease in an elderly patient and may occur in the absence of any clinical signs usually associated with acute cholecystitis.

Diagnosis. The diagnosis of acute cholecystitis should be considered in any elderly patient with documented gallstone disease who has right upper quadrant pain lasting for more than 12 hours, regardless of the presence of fever or an elevated white blood cell count. Furthermore, the diagnosis of acute cholecystitis should be pursued in the elderly patient who presents with sepsis of undetermined etiology.[77] Rapid diagnosis and implementation of appropriate therapy are essential.

Liver function tests

Other than demonstrating an elevated white blood cell count, routine laboratory evaluation may be of little benefit for most patients. However, the increased incidence of choledocholithiasis, which has been well-documented in the elderly, suggests that liver function tests may be of greater benefit in the geriatric population. This is underscored by the fact that jaundice is a major finding in many elderly patients with symptomatic gallstone disease. Recent data from Japan indicate a significant alteration in serum tests of liver function in older patients undergoing cholecystectomy compared with their younger counterparts.[78]

Ultrasonography

Oral cholecystography has been largely replaced by abdominal ultrasonography. This eliminates the need for radiation exposure and normal intestinal absorption, hepatic secretion, and gallbladder concentration of dye, and often provides additional information about the anatomy of the bile duct and pancreas. Additionally, the procedure can be performed rapidly in an acutely ill patient. Biliary scintigraphy has not proven to be especially helpful in most patients because documentation of stones is typically sufficient to diagnose acute cholecystitis in a patient with fairly straightforward symptomatology. However, biliary scintigraphy may be helpful in the elderly patient with an atypical clinical presentation, and in whom confirmation of the diagnosis may require documentation of cystic duct occlusion.

Gram-negative aerobes and anaerobes

Treatment. The reported incidence of positive bile cultures in patients under 50 years of age is 30%, increasing to more than 50% in patients 70 years of age or older.[79] Most bacteria are of enteric origin, with *Escherichia coli* being most common. Elderly patients with acute cholecystitis require a therapeutic course of antibiotics and should not be treated merely with a prophylactic regimen. We recommend coverage for gram-negative aerobes, anaerobes, and *Enterococcus.*

Regardless of age, surgical removal of the gallbladder remains the mainstay of therapy and the only means of achieving a cure for patients with acute cholecystitis. The mortality associated with cholecystectomy for acute cholecystitis in patients over the age of 60 years is nearly ten times higher than that in younger patients. However, current death rates are appreciably lower than those reported previously, in part because of underlying medical conditions and improved parasurgical care.

Although open cholecystectomy has been the treatment of choice for many years, the emergence of laparoscopic cholecystectomy has provided an interesting and attractive option. In three series describing more than 1,000 patients undergoing laparoscopic cholecystectomy, only 57 patients were thought to have acute cholecystitis.[80-82] In this combined series the success rate ranged from 40% to 70%, with a corresponding conversion rate of 5% to 60%. No major complications were reported. This latter finding probably reflects the operators' expertise and willingness to convert to an open procedure. Laparoscopic cholecystectomy can be performed safely in patients with acute cholecystitis, but it should not be undertaken until the surgeon has had sufficient experience with more routine cases. These principles have been well articulated in a recent report of 25 patients with acute cholecystitis who underwent laparoscopic cholecystectomy with no significant morbidity and mortality.[83] Regardless of individual experience, one should have a low threshold for converting to an open procedure. The experience with laparoscopic cholecystectomy in this setting is limited, and there are no available data focusing on the elderly. However, minimally invasive surgery may be perfectly appropriate and even desirable when it can be performed in this setting without any additional risk or mortality. It is important to reemphasize the concept that the underlying cardiovascular status of the patient rather than the biliary disease, per se, will determine the outcome of cholecystectomy.

Conversion to an open procedure may be necessary

Cholecystostomy has been advocated for certain high-risk individuals and generally can be performed with the patient under local anesthesia.[84] Cholecystostomy may convert a potentially grave medical situation to a managable one. The usual indication for cholecystostomy is a serious hepatic, cardiovascular, or pulmonary disorder in a critically ill patient who has developed acute cholecystitis. Recognizing the high incidence of choledocholithiasis in the geriatric population, it is essential to document radiographically the patency of the cystic duct in any elderly patient undergoing cholecystostomy. Depending on the patient's circumstances, the presence of common duct calculi may not mandate common bile duct exploration. Cholecystostomy provides access to the biliary tract, and asymptomatic common duct stones may be removed subsequently using radiologic or endoscopic techniques. The overall operative mortality from cholecystostomy varies between 25% and 40%. This high mortality relative to cholecystectomy probably reflects the severe medical diseases of the elderly patient rather than the selection of the operation itself.

Cholecystostomy for the high-risk elderly patient

Recent interest has focused on ultrasound-guided percutaneous transhepatic cholecystostomy[85] and endoscopic transpapillary drainage of the gallbladder as alternatives to surgical cholecystostomy.[86] This technology is potentially very interesting, particularly as a therapeutic modality in the elderly, but the safety and efficacy of these procedures remain to be defined.

Choledocholithiasis

Common bile duct stones have been reported in 20% to 54% of elderly patients undergoing cholecystectomy, but in less than 15% of younger patients. Although the exact reason for this difference has never been elucidated, most authorities believe that it reflects physician attitudes and a natural reluctance to recommend elective surgery in the elderly. The clinical impact of the increased incidence of choledocholithiasis in this population is underscored by the mortality associated with common bile duct exploration, which increases with age: 0.9% in patients less than 50 years of age[87] and 7% to 29% in patients more than 70 years of age.[88]

Special considerations in the elderly argue for conservative surgery

There are a number of perplexing issues related to the management of common duct stones in the elderly, primarily intraoperative management, the rationale for protective or prophylactic biliary-enteric bypass, and the role of preoperative ERCP and sphincterotomy. A number of authors have recommended that choledochoduodenostomy be considered in any elderly patient with multiple common bile duct stones[87,89] because of the difficulty in stone extraction in some patients and the low morbidity and mortality associated with this type of bypass. It has been our policy not to proceed with prophylactic bypass unless there is a clear-cut indication, such as many retained stones, recurrent or primary stones, bile duct abnormalities, or strictures. The ability of radiologists to basket the stones, and of endoscopists to perform sphincterotomy, has led us to recommend doing only what is necessary at the time of

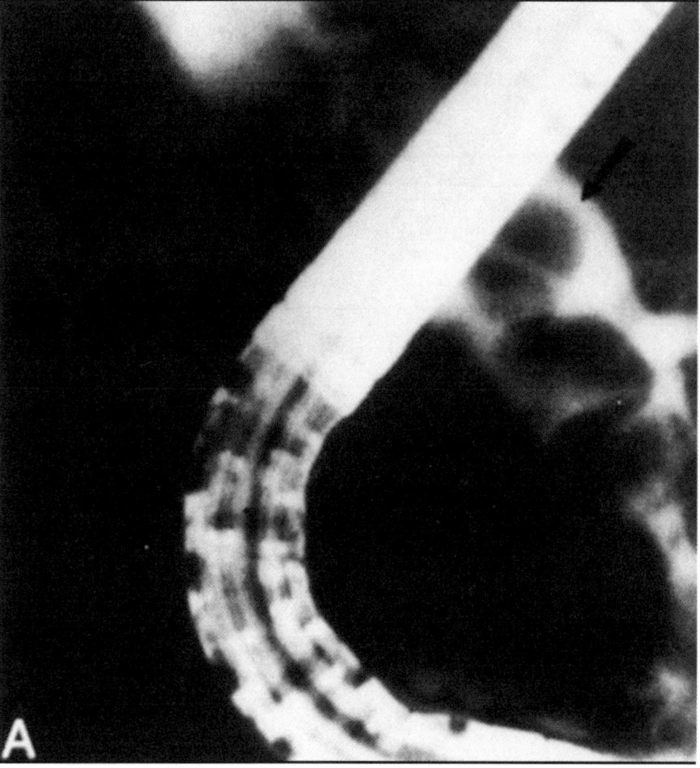

Fig. 2. ERCP demonstrating multiple common bile duct calculi in an 81-year-old man. Endoscopic sphincterotomy was performed prior to cholecystectomy.

laparotomy. In general, the acutely ill geriatric patient should undergo a meticulous and expeditious operation that provides the greatest chance of cure with the least risk.

Figure 2

Preoperative ERCP and sphincterotomy prior to open or laparoscopic cholecystectomy has proved useful in the management of patients with suspected common bile duct stones.[90,91] This procedure can be performed safely with minimal morbidity and mortality, and may obviate the need for a protracted and lengthy operation and facilitate a laparoscopic cholecystectomy, which otherwise may not be thought feasible (Fig. 2). Additional data suggest that this approach may be more cost-effective than conventional management strategies.[90] It would reduce operative time, perhaps eliminate the need for laparotomy, and facilitate the perioperative care of the frail elderly.

Perforation

Table 3

In some elderly, gallbladder ischemia may lead to perforation

It has long been recognized that perforation of the gallbladder occurs more frequently among the aged than among the young (Table 3). Recent data suggest that this clinical observation may be a consequence of circulatory changes in the elderly, rendering the least well vascularized portion of the gallbladder ischemic. This hypothesis is supported by the finding that the fundus is the most common site of gallbladder perforation.[92] The most common type of perforation is type III, in which there is a fistula between the gallbladder and a segment of the gastrointestinal tract, typically the duodenum. Type I (acute perforation with bile duct peritonitis) and type II (subacute perforation with pericholecystic abscess) occur less frequently, but are equally challenging to manage.

Although gallstone ileus is a relatively rare condition that accounts for less than 5% of intestinal obstructions in the general population, it is of some importance in the elderly.

Table 3. Clinical Profiles Associated With Gallbladder Perforation

	Type I (Acute Perforation With Bile Duct Peritonitis)	Type III (Chronic Perforation With Cholecystoenteric Fistula)
Gender	Male > Female	Male = Female
Age	Young	Elderly
History of biliary disease	No	Yes
Onset	Acute	Insidious

Modified from Roslyn and Thompson.[92]

Gallstone ileus and small-bowel obstruction

Gallstone ileus is responsible for 20% to 25% of cases of small-bowel obstruction in elderly women.[93] Frequently the stone becomes impacted in the terminal ileum, and the presentation is typical of a distal small-bowel obstruction. The diagnosis is often suggested by the finding of air within the intrahepatic biliary tract on plain abdominal radiographs. Palpation of a stone in the small bowel at the time of laparotomy confirms the diagnosis. Attention should be focused initially on relief of the mechanical small-bowel obstruction by proximal enterotomy and stone removal. Takedown of the biliary-enteric fistula and cholecystectomy should be considered at the time of the initial laparotomy if there is evidence of acute biliary tract disease or if the cholecystectomy could be performed easily without subjecting the patient to inordinate risk.

Emphysematous Cholecystitis

Gas-forming bacteria

Acute emphysematous cholecystitis is an unusual clinical entity that is characterized by the radiographic demonstration of gas within the gallbladder lumen or wall. It is more common in elderly men and diabetics, and is associated with gangrene and perforation of the gallbladder. Clostridial organisms are present in most patients with emphysematous cholecystitis, although other gas-forming organisms may be found as well. The pathogenesis of this disorder is not clear, although gallstones are absent in up to 50% of patients. Ischemia has been implicated as a potential etiologic factor in this process. The associated mortality is high, and prompt cholecystectomy is indicated.

Cancer

Carcinomas of the gallbladder and extrahepatic biliary tract are an uncommon form of gastrointestinal malignancy. They are present in less than 10% of colorectal cancer patients in the United States of America and tend to occur in older patients. Curative resection for gallbladder or bile duct tumors is infrequent, and these lesions continue to present a formidable challenge to the surgeon. The diagnosis of gallbladder carcinoma is typically made during or following cholecystectomy. More so than for most gastrointestinal malignancies, the treatment of extrahepatic biliary tract carcinoma typically includes a multidisciplinary approach employing endoscopic, radiologic, and surgical expertise.

Predominantly a disease of women

Gallbladder Cancer. Carcinoma of the gallbladder is the most common cancer involving the hepatobiliary tract and accounts for approximately two thirds of cancers of the extrahepatic biliary tract. The association between cholelithiasis and carcinoma of the gallbladder has been well described.[94] Therefore, it is not surprising that carcinoma of the gallbladder is predominantly a disease of women (the female-to-male ratio is between 3:1 and 5:1). Although the vast majority of patients with carcinoma of the gallbladder have gallstones, the converse is not true and, in fact, the incidence of gallbladder cancer is quite low among patients with cholelithiasis.

Typically, the diagnosis of gallbladder carcinoma is made during cholecystectomy performed for symptomatic chole-

Gallbladder carcinoma recognized at laparotomy

lithiasis. Although surgical extirpation of the gallbladder and surrounding tissues continues to be the mainstay of treatment for patients with gallbladder carcinoma, the ideal treatment for patients with gallbladder tumors recognized at laparotomy, or individuals in whom the diagnosis is made postoperatively during pathologic examination of the specimen, remains unclear.[95] These issues become even more complicated in elderly patients. Recommendations vary widely, and range from simple cholecystectomy to cholecystectomy with regional lymphadenectomy and wedge resection of the gallbladder bed to more radical procedures, including resection of the right hepatic lobe and medial segment of the left lobe.[96-98] The long-term benefits of such radical procedures for patients with carcinoma of the gallbladder continue to be an area of investigation, but such procedures are probably not warranted in the elderly, because the only curable lesions are those that are removed incidentally during cholecystectomy. It has been our practice to proceed with regional lymphadenectomy and wedge resection of the liver in cases in which an intraoperative diagnosis of resectable gallbladder carcinoma has been made definitively. This should be considered only in low-risk patients if the surgeon feels that this additional procedure will not add substantially to morbidity or mortality.

Gallbladder carcinoma recognized postoperatively

A more difficult issue involves the individual in whom the diagnosis of gallbladder carcinoma is confirmed postoperatively. Should such a patient be reoperated on and undergo lymphadenectomy and some form of hepatic resection? This question has not been resolved. Patients with stage I disease, in whom the tumor is intramucosal, have probably been treated adequately by total cholecystectomy. Nonetheless, a more aggressive posture to such a patient would not be unwarranted and should be considered in patients with stage II disease where the tumor is submucosal, or stage III disease where the tumor is serosal.

For a bile duct cancer—Surgical extirpation vs nonsurgical management

Bile Duct Cancer. Carcinoma of the extrahepatic biliary tract is a relatively uncommon malignancy that appears on 0.01% to 0.5% of autopsies. Carcinoma of the bile duct tends to be a disease of the elderly, with a mean age at presentation between 60 and 65 years in most reported series. In one recent series of 186 patients with documented bile duct cancers, 23% of the patients were over the age of 70 years.[99] Although surgical extirpation provides the only chance for cure in these patients,[100,101] recent studies advocate the nonsurgical management of malignant biliary obstruction using biliary endoprostheses placed endoscopically or via the percutaneous transhepatic route.[102,103] Nonoperative biliary decompression has been advocated for the treatment of elderly patients in whom results of radiographic studies indicate a lack of tumor resectability (Fig. 3). Advantages to nonoperative management for elderly patients with bile duct tumors include shorter initial hospital stays, a lower incidence of procedure-related morbidity, and a 30-day mortality of 9% to 15%. In a more recent review of 42 consecutive patients over the age of 70 years with a confirmed histologic diagnosis of bile duct cancer who were treated at a single institution, the 30-day mortality was only 10%.[99]

Figure 3

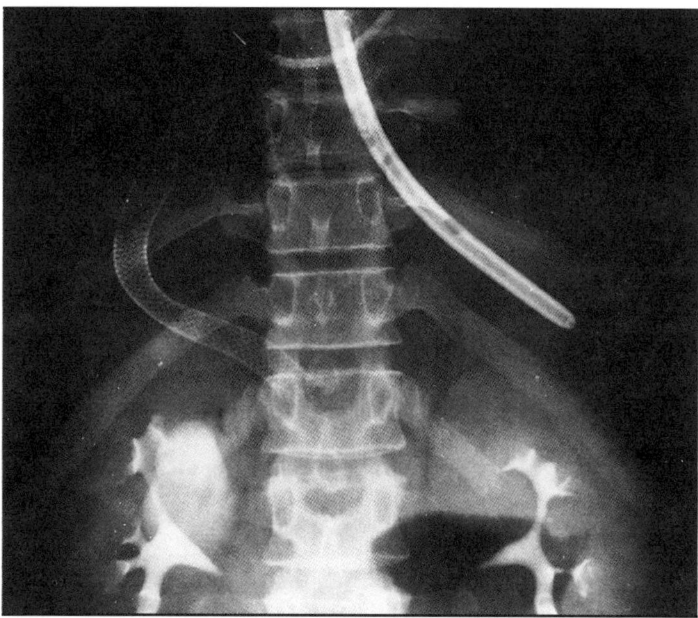

Fig. 3. Plain abdominal x-ray demonstrating a metallic prosthesis placed by a radiologist to stent a malignant biliary obstruction in a 76-year-old woman with unresectable carcinoma.

Nonoperative management has several potential disadvantages that also need to be considered. A definitive histologic or cytologic diagnosis is not obtained in approximately 70% of patients.[104] Furthermore, the lack of tumor resectability is established via indirect radiographic means. Even with the sophisticated cholangiographic techniques currently available, bile duct tumors (which tend to be small focal adenocarcinomas) can be difficult to diagnose radiographically, and even harder to stage. Finally, two recent studies suggest that nonoperative decompression may be associated with a poorer quality of life than operative decompression when factors such as frequency of hospital readmission, incidence of catheter-related problems, and postprocedural pain and jaundice are taken into account.[105,106] There is little question that nonoperatively placed biliary prostheses play a role in the treatment of elderly patients with bile duct tumors, particularly those who are not surgical candidates based on their degree of comor-bidity. However, recent surgical data indicate that the operative management of bile duct tumors in elderly patients provides an opportunity for a definitive diagnosis, which can be established in 95% of cases.[99]

Operative management yields definite diagnosis

PANCREATIC DISEASE

Anatomic and functional changes occur in the aging pancreas. Total weight of the gland has been shown to decrease after the age of 70 years, with a loss of approximately 15% by the age of 85 years.[107] Histologic changes associated with aging include fatty replacement of pancreatic lobules and fibrosis in a patchy manner without extensive loss of exocrine parenchyma.[107] Proliferation of ductal epithelium with subsequent recanalization and expansion of obliterated ducts results in cystic cavitation.[108] In addition to these histologic changes, progressive duct ectasia is also noted on pancreatography in association with advancing age.[109] Although functional changes such as decreased exocrine responses to secretin and CCK have been observed with aging, the clinical significance of these alterations remains unclear.[110,111]

Pancreatitis

Although there does not appear to be any greater propensity for elderly patients to develop acute pancreatitis, the epidemiology of this disorder is different in older patients than in younger patients. The more common causes of acute pancreatitis in the geriatric population include gallstones, medications, metabolic derangements, tumors, and ischemia.[112] Alcoholic pancreatitis is seen much less commonly in older patients for reasons that are unclear. The incidence of acute pancreatitis is equivalent in men and women below the age of 50 years. However, elderly women have a greater incidence of pancreatitis than do elderly men.[113] This trend is probably indicative of the increased incidence of biliary pancreatitis in this age group. The mortality associated with acute pancreatitis in the elderly is significantly higher than that in the general population. Cornfield et al[114] reported a 28% mortality among acute pancreatitis patients over the age of 60 years compared with a 9% mortality among younger acute pancreatitis patients. Similar findings have been reported by other authors.[113]

Acute pancreatitis and elderly women

Biliary Pancreatitis. In elderly patients with biliary pancreatitis the timing and method of intervention is absolutely critical. Although treatment options may vary, a goal for all elderly patients with gallstone pancreatitis should be the implementation of definitive therapy prior to discharge. This proposal is based on the 30% to 40% recurrence rate of acute pancreatitis in patients who are discharged from the hospital without their underlying processes having been corrected. Ultimately, the goals of any therapy should be to clear the common bile duct of residual stones and, ideally, remove the gallbladder to prevent any further complications of cholelithiasis.

A high recurrence rate mandates definite therapy

Traditional teaching has suggested that cholecystectomy and intraoperative cholangiography should be performed in patients who are good operative risks and who experience prompt resolution of their pancreatic inflammation. Common bile duct exploration should be performed based on intraoperative and cholangiographic findings. Early surgery (prior to the resolution of acute pancreatitis) has been advocated by some, but most surgeons prefer to allow resolution of the pancreatitis prior to exploration.[114,115] Data from two separate randomized studies comparing conventional surgery alone with preoperative sphincterotomy followed by surgery failed to demonstrate any significant benefit of the combined approach.[116,117] An interesting analysis of 173 patients with choledocholithiasis has indicated that endoscopic stone removal immediately prior to cholecystectomy may be more cost-effective than cholecystectomy and common bile duct exploration.[118] Adherence to this approach may allow the performance of a laparoscopic cholecystectomy in a patient who otherwise would require open operation.

Is subsequent cholecystectomy mandatory in a patient with biliary pancreatitis who undergoes a successful ERCP and sphincterotomy? Recent data suggest that the incidence of recurrent symptoms will be minimal in the vast majority of patients, and elective cholecystectomy will not be required.[119,120] The application of this finding as it relates to the elderly is considerable.

The importance of endoscopic sphincterotomy in the management of severe gallstone pancreatitis is now well recognized, resulting in reduced morbidity, hospital stay, and mortality.[121]

Medications as causative factors

Drug-Related Pancreatitis. A variety of medications frequently administered to elderly patients have been implicated as possible factors in the development of acute pancreatitis. These include thiazides, sulfonamides, tetracyclines, valproic acid, 6-mercaptopurine, and L-asparaginase,[122] as well as ethacrynic acid, corticosteroids, chlorthalidone, and metronidazole.[123]

After surgical trauma

Postoperative Pancreatitis. Operative trauma has been cited as the second most common cause of pancreatitis in the geriatric population.[112] Clinical experience suggests that this complication, which is associated with significant morbidity and mortality, can occur after biliary procedures, gastric or esophageal resections, colectomies, splenectomies, and aortic reconstruction.

Adenocarcinoma

Pancreatitis Associated With Carcinoma. A relatively uncommon cause of acute pancreatitis, even in the elderly, is adenocarcinoma of the pancreas. Presumably this complication results from ductal obstruction.

Ischemia after hemorrhagic or other shock

Ischemia-Induced Pancreatitis. Pancreatitis is thought to also develop as a result of low flow during shock or cardiopulmonary bypass. Acute pancreatitis has been reported to occur in up to 50% of patients presenting with ruptured abdominal aortic aneurysms who develop oliguric shock.[124] In 1976, Feiner reported that 20% of patients who die following cardiac surgery have histologic evidence of acute pancreatitis.[125] The histologic pattern noted suggests that ischemia is the key element initiating pancreatitis in this setting.[126]

Complications. Geriatric patients with acute pancreatitis are particularly prone to pulmonary complications and colonic ischemia.[127] Older patients have been shown to develop pulmonary complications such as left-side pleural effusion, atelectasis, and pneumonia up to three times more frequently than are younger patients.[128]

Pseudocysts

The most common complication of acute pancreatitis is the development of pseudocysts. If symptomatic, drainage is advocated. For mature pseudocysts, internal drainage is considered preferable to external drainage because of the latter's higher potential for pseudocyst recurrence and pancreatic fistulas. Preoperative ERCP may be helpful by evaluating the pancreatic duct and its relation to the pseudocyst. Drainage of a dilated, obstructed pancreatic duct often can be performed easily at the time of cyst enterostomy.

In the geriatric patient with concurrent disease, the risk of an operative approach may be prohibitive. Growing experience with percutaneous and transgastric drainage of pseudocysts indicates the feasibility of these nonoperative approaches, although the indications, complications, and limitations of these approaches have not been defined completely.

The necessity for treatment of asymptomatic pseudocysts is controversial. Some have advocated an expectant approach based on recent experience indicating that the potential complications of infection, hemorrhage, and rupture have not occurred. An additional consideration, especially in the geriatric patient, is the possibility of cystic neoplasms. Although cystadenomas characteristically occur in middle-aged women, there have been sporadic reports of this diagnosis in geriatric patients. Cystadenocarcinomas are rare but classically seen in the elderly. In the older patient who is a suitable candidate for general anesthesia and laparotomy, an operative approach allows the establishment of a definitive diagnosis by cyst wall biopsy. The appropriate operative procedure can then be performed.

Chronic Pancreatitis. Chronic pancreatitis is the second most common cause of steatorrhea in the elderly. Although it is usually associated with chronic abdominal pain, chronic pancreatitis may be painless in 5% to 15% of cases.[129] Pancreatic carcinoma is the most important differential diagnosis to consider in the elderly patient presenting with abdominal pain and the nutritional deficiencies resulting from protein and fat malabsorption.

Management options in chronic pancreatitis

The treatment of chronic pain depends on its severity and the extent to which the patient is debilitated. Nonoperative therapy for mild to moderate pain has been predicated on the observation that up to 50% of patients report a lessening of pain intensity over the course of at least 5 years. Theoretically, this effect is due to negative feedback regulation of pancreatic secretion by intraduodenal trypsin. In the presence of a dilated pancreatic duct, operative drainage procedures are highly successful in relieving pain. Classically, the pancreatic duct is obstructed by multiple strictures resulting in the "chain-of-lakes" appearance on ERCP, necessitating lateral pancreaticojejunostomy (Puestow's procedure) for complete drainage. When a single stricture exists in the proximal duct, distal pancreatectomy with end pancreaticojejunostomy (Duvall's procedure) should drain the obstructed pancreatic duct adequately. However, recent experience with this procedure has been less than optimal. Overall, drainage procedures are successful in alleviating pain in up to 80% of cases; the associated mortality is less than 2%. Recent experience supports the use of earlier drainage, before end-stage chronic pancreatitis and debilitating pain have developed. Management decisions should be based on the nature of the intrinsic pancreatic disease and the patient's overall medical status, not age alone.

Early drainage

Cancer

The incidence of cancer of the pancreas is 50 times higher in patients 80 to 84 years of age than in patients 40 to 44 years of age. Pancreatic cancer now represents the fourth most common cause of cancer and, thus, cannot be regarded as an uncommon problem in the elderly. Nevertheless, the diagnosis of pancreatic cancer is usually made at an advanced stage due to its early nonspecific clinical presentation. Useful studies when the diagnosis is suspected include CT, ultrasound and, most recently, endoscopic ultrasound. Further evaluation of a periampullary mass is made by ERCP, during which biopsies of the ampulla, brushings of the biliary tree, and cytology of aspirated pancreatic and biliary secretions can establish the diagnosis in most patients.

The decision to proceed with surgery for pancreatic cancer is a complex one. An important determination is the resectability of the disease. In the presence of metastases, malignant ascites, or gross local extension, palliation by nonoperative means is probably advisable. The therapeutic decision is more difficult in the patient with a potentially resectable lesion. In these cases, routine arteriography has been recommended by some for staging purposes. When extensive, vessel encasement generally indicates unresectability. However, vessel encasement to a lesser degree has not been reliable in predicting unresectability in patients who have been explored subsequently. Routine angiography also has been advocated for the detection of anatomic aberrations; however, these are usually evident intraoperatively. Angiography has not been used routinely in our approach to elderly patients who are being considered for curative resection.

Factors influencing the therapeutic decision

Laparoscopy is another procedure that may be useful in the staging process, as it can detect metastatic lesions smaller than the resolution of CT. However, this procedure is of value only if the detection of metastatic disease alters the subsequent approach to palliation.

In the past, surgical palliation was the only option for biliary obstruction due to unresectable carcinoma of the pancreas. The introduction of percutaneous and endoscopic techniques for stent placement has prompted a reevaluation of management strategies for these patients. In the elderly, many of whom have reason to avoid general anesthesia and the risks of an operative procedure, endoscopic stent placement may be a better option for palliating biliary obstruction. However, duodenal obstruction still requires surgical bypass by gastroenterostomy. Biliary drainage may be performed as part of the operative procedure unless local extension of the primary precludes access to the extrahepatic biliary tree.

Resectable pancreatic cancer

For patients with resectable pancreatic cancers, operative mortality has decreased and long-term survival has increased since the early experience with the Whipple procedure. Recent reports indicate less than a 5% mortality associated with pancreaticoduodenectomy in certain centers. This has been attributed to increasing experience with the procedure, technical modifications of the resection, and new methods of treating leaks from the pancreatic anastomosis. The management of leaks from the pancreaticojejunostomy has been facilitated by the introduction of octreotide. This analogue of somatostatin effectively suppresses pancreatic exocrine excretion. A once-dreaded complication can now be managed more easily and, perhaps, avoided.

Improvement in long-term survival following curative resec-

Age alone is no barrier to pancreatic resection

tion alone also has been reported. In addition, the chances for long-term survival have been enhanced by adjuvant chemotherapy and radiotherapy. Thus, in an appropriately selected group of patients with resectable disease, curative resection can be performed with a relatively low operative mortality and increased long-term survival. Age greater than 65 years is no longer considered a contraindication to radical pancreatic resection.

The approach to pancreatic cancer must be individualized. The chance for a curative resection must be balanced by a realistic assessment of risk and longevity with particular recognition that limited treatment cannot be justified on the basis of age alone.

References

1. Reiss R, Deutsch AA. *J Gerontol* 1985;40:154-158.
2. Huber DF, et al. *Am J Surg* 1983;146:719-722.
3. Morrow DJ, et al. *Arch Surg* 1978;113:1149-1152.
4. Ibach JR Jr, et al. *Surg Gynecol Obstet* 1968;126:523-528.
5. Glenn F, Hays DM. *Surg Gynecol Obstet* 1955;100:11-18.
6. Krarup T, et al. *Acta Chir Scand* 1982;148:263-266.
7. McSherry CK, Glenn F. *Ann Surg* 1980;191:271-275.
8. McSherry CK, et al. *Ann Surg* 1985;202:59-63.
9. Wait RB, Kahng KU. *Am J Surg* 1989;157:256-263.
10. James OFW. *Clin Gastroenterol* 1983;12:671-691.
11. Okuda K, et al, in Kitank (ed). *Liver and Aging.* Amsterdam, North Holland, Elsevier, 1978, pp 159-176.
12. Mooney H, et al. *Clin Gastroenterol* 1985;14:757-771.
13. Watanabe T, Tanaka Y. *Virchows Arch* 1982;39:9-20.
14. Kampmann JP, et al. *Geriatrics* 1975;30:91-95.
15. Koff RRS, et al. *Gastroenterology* 1973;65:300-302.
16. Woodhouse KW. *Clin Gastroenterol* 1985;14:863-880.
17. Bateson MC. *Lancet* 1984;2:621.
18. Bowen JC, et al. *Med Clin North Am* 1992;76:1143-1157.
19. Lise M, et al. *Dis Colon Rectum* 1990;33:688-694.
20. Registry of Hepatic Metastases. *Surgery* 1988;103:278-288.
21. Asbun HJ, Hughes KS. *Surg Clin North Am* 1993;73:165-166.
22. Roslyn JJ, et al. *Arch Surg* 1984;119:1312-1315.
23. Linsell A, in Wanebo HJ (ed). *Hepatic and Biliary Cancer.* New York, Marcel Dekker, Inc, 1987, p 4.
24. Chen J-C, et al. *Radiology* 1984;150:797.
25. Kuntslinger F, et al. *Am J Radiol* 1980;134:431.
26. Clouse ME. *Surg Clin North Am* 1993;69:193-234.
27. Adson MA, Weiland LH. *Am J Surg* 1981;141:18-21.
28. Jwatsuki S, et al. *Ann Surg* 1983;197:247-252.
29. Sesto ME, et al. *Surgery* 1987;102:846-851.
30. Ezaki T, et al. *Br J Surg* 1987;74:471-473.
31. Gyorffy EJ, et al. *Ann Surg* 1987;206:699-705.
32. Gerzof SG, et al. *Am J Surg* 1985;149:487-494.
33. Ferrucci JT, van Sonnenberg E. *JAMA* 1980;246:487-494.
34. Khalil T, et al. *Surgery* 1985;98:423-429.
35. Floyd JC, et al. *Recent Prog Horm Res* 1977;33:519-570.
36. Conter RL, et al. *Gastroenterology* 1987;92:771-776.
37. Heaton KW. *Clin Gastroenterol* 1973;2:67-83.
38. Lieber MM. *Ann Surg* 1952;135:394-405.
39. Friedman GD, et al. *J Chronis Dis* 1966;19:273-292.
40. Glenn F. *Ann Surg* 1981;193:56-59.
41. Krarup T, et al. *Acta Clin Scand* 1982;148:263-266.
42. Mentzer RM, et al. *Am J Surg* 1975;129:10-15.
43. Rosly JJ, et al. *Am J Gastro* 1987;82:636-640.
44. Norman DC, Yoshikawa TT. *J Am Geratr Soc* 1983;31:677-684.
45. Reiss R, et al. *World J Surg* 1990;14:567-571.
46. Gililand TM, Traverso W. *Am J Surg* 1990;159:489-492.
47. Ransohoff DF, Gracie WA. *Am J Med* 1990;88:154-160.
48. Schreiber H, et al. *Am J Surg* 1978;135:196-198.

49. Quiriel K, et al. *Ann Surg* 1983;198:717-719.
50. Johnson LB. *Surg Gynecol Obstet* 1987;164:197-203.
51. Roslyn JJ, et al. *Ann Surg,* to be published.
52. Glenn F. *Surg Gynecol Obstet* 1975;140:877-884.
53. Herzog U, et al. *Surg Gynecol Obstet* 1992;175:238-242.
54. Dubois F, et al. *Ann Surg* 1990;211:609-612.
55. Schirmer BD, et al. *Ann Surg* 1991;213:665-677.
56. The Southern Surgeon's Club. *N Engl J Med* 1991;324:1073-1078.
57. Airan M, et al. *Surg Endoscop* 1992;6:169-176.
58. Litwin DEM, et al. *Can J Surg* 1992;35:291-296.
59. Stockmann PT, et al. *Arch Surg* 1992;127:917-923.
60. Cusschieri A, et al. *Am J Surg* 1991;161:385-387.
61. Dent TL. *Am J Surg* 1991;161:399-403.
62. Peters JH, et al. *Surgery* 1991;110:769-777.
63. Ponsky JL. *Am J Surg* 1991;161:393-395.
64. Nenner RP, et al. *NY State J Med* 1992;92:179-181.
65. Wittgen CM, et al. *Arch Surg* 1991;126:997-1000.
66. Delman GR, et al. *Br J Anaesth* 1972;44:1155-1162.
67. Schoenfield LJ, et al. *Ann Intern Med* 1981;95:257-281.
68. Weinstein MC, et al. *J Gen Intern Med* 1990;5:277-284.
69. Thistle JF, et al. *N Engl J Med* 1989;320:633-639.
70. Sackmann M, et al. *N Engl J Med* 1988;318:393-397.
71. Herberer G, et al. *Ann Surg* 1988;208:274-278.
72. Magnuson TH, et al. *Arch Surg* 1989;124:1195-1201.
73. Bass EB, et al. *Gastroenterology* 1991;101:189-199.
74. Saunders-Kirkwood K, et al. *Ann Surg* 1992;215:318-325.
75. Hafif A, et al. *Am Surg* 1991; 57:648-652.
76. Cobden I, et al. *Lancet* 1984;1:1062-1064.
77. Madden JW, et al. *Postgrad Med J* 1981;57:502-506.
78. Shinagawa N, et al. *Jap J Surg* 1992;22:29-34.
79. Shimada K, et al. *J Clin Infect Dis* 1977;135:850-854.
80. Graves HA, et al. *Ann Surg* 1991;213:655-662.
81. Reddick EJ, et al. *Am J Surg* 1991;214:531-540.
82. Bailey RW, et al. *Ann Surg* 1991;214:531-540.
83. Phillips EH, et al. *Am Surg* 1992;58:273-276.
84. Kaufman M, et al. *Surg Gynecol Obstet* 1990; 170:533-537.
85. McGahan JP, et al. *Radiology* 1989;173:481-485.
86. Feretis CB, et al. *Gastrointest Endoscop* 1990;36:523-525.
87. Haff FC, et al. *Arch Surg* 1969;98:428-434.
88. Lygidakis NJ. *Surg Gynecol Obstet* 1983;157:15-19.
89. Moesgaard F, et al. *Surg Gynecol Obstet* 1982;154:232-234.
90. Stiegmann G, et al. *Arch Surg* 1989;124:787-790.
91. Boulay J, et al. *Am J Gastro* 1992;87:837-842.
92. Roslyn JJ, et al. *Am J Gastro* 1987;82:636-640.
93. Cooperman AM, et al. *Ann Surg* 1968;377-383.
94. Diehl AK. *JAMA* 1983;250:2323-2326.
95. Bergdahl L. *Ann Surg* 1980;191:19-22.
96. Nakamura S, et al. *Surgery* 1989;106:467-473.
97. Ouchi K, et al. *Surgery* 1987;101:731-737.
98. Silk YN, et al. *Ann Surg* 1989;210:751-757.
99. Saunders K, et al. *Arch Surg* 1991;126:1186-1191.
100. Bismuth H, et al. *World J Surg* 1988;12:39-47.
101. Cameron JL, et al. *Am J Surg* 1990;159:91-98.
102. Speer AG, et al. *Lancet* 1987;2:57-62.
103. Shepherd HA, et al. *Br J Surg* 1988;75:1166-1168.
104. Saunders K, et al. *Arch Surg* 1991;126:1186-1191.
105. Lai ECS, et al. *Ann Surg* 1987;205:111-118.
106. Lai ECS, et al. *Am J Surg* 1992;163:208-212.
107. Rossle O. *Beitraege zur pathologischen Anatomie und zur Allgemeinen Pathologie* 1921;163:69-79.
108. Andrew W. *Am J Anat* 1944;74:97-127.
109. Kreel L, Sandin B. *Gut* 1973;14:962-970.
110. Rosenberg IR, et al. *Gastroenterology* 1966;50:191-194.
111. Langier R, Sarles H. *Clin Gastroenterol* 1985;14:749-756.
112. Park J, et al. *Am J Surg* 1986;152:638-642.
113. Hoffman E, et al. *Gastroenterology* 1959;36:675.
114. Cornfield AP, et al. *Gut* 1985;26:724-729.
115. Stone HH, et al. *Ann Surg* 1981;194:305-312.
116. Neoptolemos JP, et al. *Br J Surg* 1987;294:470-474.
117. Tsuchiyose M, et al. *Gastroenterology* 1989;96:A516.

118. van Stiegman G, et al. *Arch Surg* 1989;124:787-789.
119. Kullman E, et al. *Eur J Surg* 1991;157:131-135.
120. Hill J, et al. *Br J Surg* 1991;78:554-556.
121. Neoptolemos JP, et al. *Lancet* 1988;2:979.
122. Mallory KA, et al. *Gastroenterology* 1980;78:813-820.
123. Sanford KA, et al. *Ann Intern Med* 1988;109:756.
124. Warshaw AL, O'Hara PJ. *Ann Surg* 1978;188:197-201.
125. Feiner H. *Am J Surg* 1976;181:684-688.
126. Foulis AK. *J Clin Pathol* 1982;35:1244.
127. Ingber S, Jacobson IM. *Gastroenterol Clin North Am* 1990;19:433-457.
128. Ranson JHC, et al. *Ann Surg* 1974;179:557-566.
129. Fitzgerald O. *Clin Gastroenterol* 1972;1:195.

Index

Page numbers in **boldface** type refer to pages on which tables or figures appear; an *italic t* or *f* denotes tables or figures, respectively.

RECENT DATA

CONFIDENCE

MEFOXIN® IV/IM

(CEFOXITIN SODIUM)

In a recent study of penetrating abdominal trauma, 144 patients (85% of total) were categorized in group 1 (low risk) and had 2 days of antibiotic therapy; 26 patients (15% of total) were categorized as group 2 or group 3 (mid or high risk) and received 5 days of antibiotic therapy.[1]

MORE EFFECTIVE THAN CEFOTAN* IN LOW-RISK PATIENTS**

...in preventing infection in 2-day therapy group

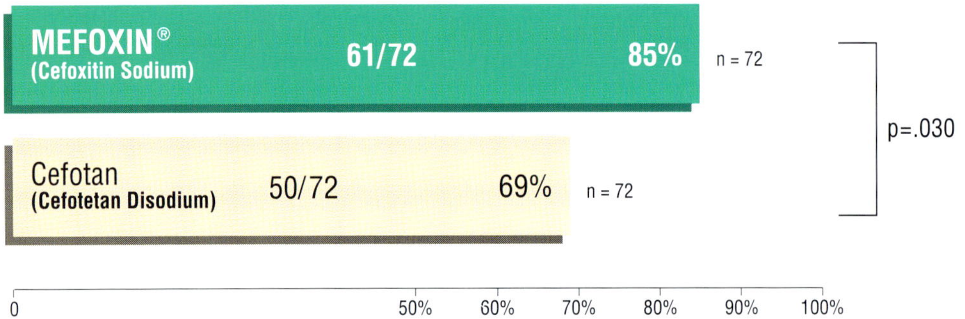

Percentage of patients remaining infection-free

...in significantly reducing length of hospital stay in 2-day, low-risk therapy group

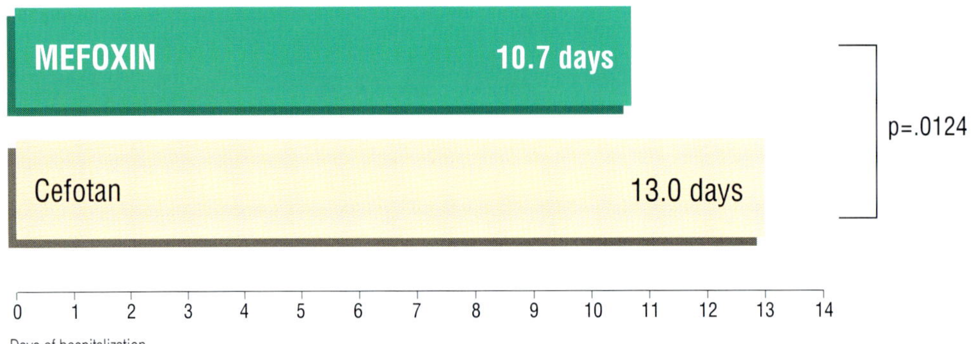

Days of hospitalization

* registered trademark of Imperial Chemical Industries PLC for cefotetan disodium

** In mid- to high-risk patients treated for 5 days, length of hospitalization was almost twice as long for cefoxitin-treated patients than for those treated with cefotetan (p=.037), while infections prevented were 47% and 36% for cefoxitin and cefotetan, respectively.

The prophylactic administration of MEFOXIN may reduce the incidence of certain postoperative infections in patients undergoing surgical procedures (e.g., hysterectomy, gastrointestinal surgery, and transurethral prostatectomy) that are classified as contaminated or potentially contaminated.

Pseudomembranous colitis, from mild to life-threatening in severity, has been reported with virtually all antibiotics (including cephalosporins); therefore, it is important to consider its diagnosis when diarrhea develops in association with antibiotic use.

1. Adapted from *Arch. Surg.*, 1993; 128:55-64

In an *in vitro** study by Goldstein and Citron[2]

A comparison of anaerobic coverage vs. Cefotan

***In vitro* susceptibilities of isolates from two community hospitals at a 32-mcg/mL breakpoint (n=215)[2]**

	*B. fragilis***	*B. thetaiota-omicron*	*B. distasonis*	*B. vulgatus*	*B. ovatus*
MEFOXIN	**97%**	**92%**	**69%**	**93%**	**82%**
Cefotan	93%	24%	16%	93%	12%

** NOTE: Based on the 1993 *Physicians' Desk Reference®*, Cefotan is usually active *in vitro* and in clinical infections against a number of organisms, including *Bacteroides* species (excluding *B. distasonis*, *B. ovatus*, and *B. thetaiotaomicron*).

MEFOXIN is contraindicated in patients who have shown hypersensitivity to cefoxitin and the cephalosporin group of antibiotics.

BEFORE THERAPY WITH 'MEFOXIN' IS INSTITUTED, CAREFUL INQUIRY SHOULD BE MADE TO DETERMINE WHETHER THE PATIENT HAS HAD PREVIOUS HYPERSENSITIVITY REACTIONS TO CEFOXITIN, CEPHALOSPORINS, PENICILLINS, OR OTHER DRUGS. THIS PRODUCT SHOULD BE GIVEN WITH CAUTION TO PENICILLIN-SENSITIVE PATIENTS. ANTIBIOTICS SHOULD BE ADMINISTERED WITH CAUTION TO ANY PATIENT WHO HAS DEMONSTRATED SOME FORM OF ALLERGY, PARTICULARLY TO DRUGS. IF AN ALLERGIC REACTION TO 'MEFOXIN' OCCURS, DISCONTINUE THE DRUG. SERIOUS HYPERSENSITIVITY REACTIONS MAY REQUIRE EPINEPHRINE AND OTHER EMERGENCY MEASURES.

* The clinical significance of these *in vitro* data has not been established.

2. Goldstein, E.J.C. and Citron, D.M., *J. Clin. Microbiol.*, 1988

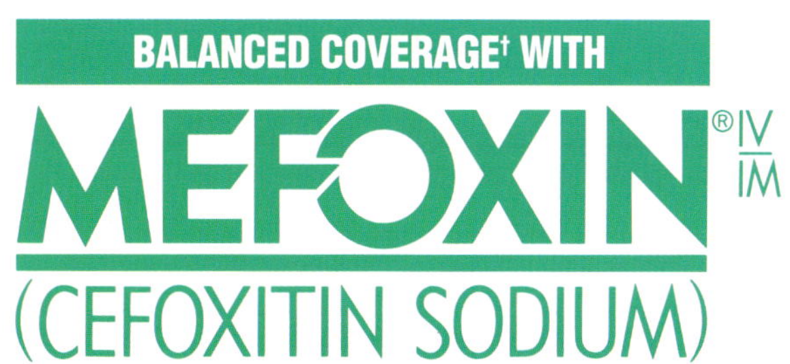

† Denotes *in vitro* activity against indicated aerobes and anaerobes. This does not necessarily imply clinical efficacy.

MEFOXIN®
(STERILE CEFOXITIN SODIUM)

DESCRIPTION

MEFOXIN* (Sterile Cefoxitin Sodium) is a semi-synthetic, broad-spectrum cepha antibiotic sealed under nitrogen for parenteral administration. It is derived from cephamycin C, which is produced by *Streptomyces lactamdurans*. It is the sodium salt of 3-(hydroxymethyl)-7α-methoxy-8-oxo-7-[2-(2-thienyl)acetamido]-5-thia-1-azabicyclo [4.2.0] oct-2-ene-2-carboxylate carbamate (ester). The empirical formula is $C_{16}H_{16}N_3NaO_7S_2$, and the structural formula is:

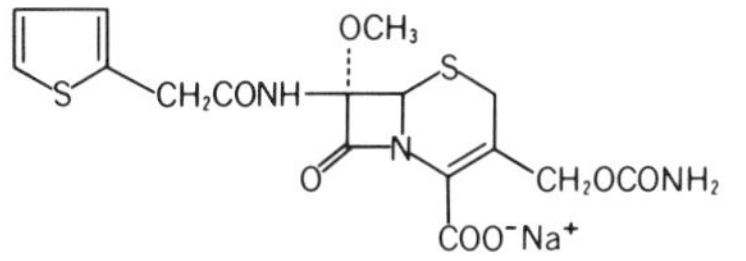

MEFOXIN contains approximately 53.8 mg (2.3 milliequivalents) of sodium per gram of cefoxitin activity. Solutions of MEFOXIN range from colorless to light amber in color. The pH of freshly constituted solutions usually ranges from 4.2 to 7.0.

CLINICAL PHARMACOLOGY

Clinical Pharmacology

After intramuscular administration of a 1 gram dose of MEFOXIN to normal volunteers, the mean peak serum concentration was 24 mcg/mL. The peak occurred at 20 to 30 minutes. Following an intravenous dose of 1 gram, serum concentrations were 110 mcg/mL at 5 minutes, declining to less than 1 mcg/mL at 4 hours. The half-life after an intravenous dose is 41 to 59 minutes; after intramuscular administration, the half-life is 64.8 minutes. Approximately 85 percent of cefoxitin is excreted unchanged by the kidneys over a 6-hour period, resulting in high urinary concentrations. Following an intramuscular dose of 1 gram, urinary concentrations greater than 3000 mcg/mL were observed. Probenecid slows tubular excretion and produces higher serum levels and increases the duration of measurable serum concentrations.

Cefoxitin passes into pleural and joint fluids and is detectable in antibacterial concentrations in bile.

Clinical experience has demonstrated that MEFOXIN can be administered to patients who are also receiving carbenicillin, kanamycin, gentamicin, tobramycin, or amikacin (see PRECAUTIONS and ADMINISTRATION).

Microbiology

The bactericidal action of cefoxitin results from inhibition of cell wall synthesis. Cefoxitin has *in vitro* activity against a wide range of gram-positive and gram-negative organisms. The methoxy group in the 7α position provides MEFOXIN with a high degree of stability in the presence of beta-lactamases, both penicillinases and cephalosporinases, of gram-negative bacteria. Cefoxitin is usually active against the following organisms *in vitro* and in clinical infections:

Gram-positive

Staphylococcus aureus, including penicillinase and non-penicillinase producing strains

*Registered trademark of MERCK & CO., INC.

MEFOXIN®
(Sterile Cefoxitin Sodium)

Staphylococcus epidermidis

Beta-hemolytic and other streptococci (most strains of enterococci, e.g., *Streptococcus faecalis,* are resistant)

Streptococcus pneumoniae

Gram-negative

Escherichia coli

Klebsiella species (including *K. pneumoniae*)

Hemophilus influenzae

Neisseria gonorrhoeae, including penicillinase and non-penicillinase producing strains

Proteus mirabilis

Morganella morganii

Proteus vulgaris

Providencia species, including *Providencia rettgeri*

Anaerobic organisms

Peptococcus species

Peptostreptococcus species

Clostridium species

Bacteroides species, including the *B. fragilis* group (includes *B. fragilis, B. distasonis, B. ovatus, B. thetaiotaomicron, B. vulgatus*)

MEFOXIN is inactive *in vitro* against most strains of *Pseudomonas aeruginosa* and enterococci and many strains of *Enterobacter cloacae.*

Methicillin-resistant staphylococci are almost uniformly resistant to MEFOXIN.

Susceptibility Tests

For fast-growing aerobic organisms, quantitative methods that require measurements of zone diameters give the most precise estimates of antibiotic susceptibility. One such procedure* has been recommended for use with discs to test susceptibility to cefoxitin. Interpretation involves correlation of the diameters obtained in the disc test with minimal inhibitory concentration (MIC) values for cefoxitin.

Reports from the laboratory giving results of the standardized single disc susceptibility test* using a 30 mcg cefoxitin disc should be interpreted according to the following criteria:

Organisms producing zones of 18 mm or greater are considered susceptible, indicating that the tested organism is likely to respond to therapy.

Organisms of intermediate susceptibility produce zones of 15 to 17 mm, indicating that the tested organism would be susceptible if high dosage is used or if the infection is confined to tissues and fluids (e.g., urine) in which high antibiotic levels are attained.

Resistant organisms produce zones of 14 mm or less, indicating that other therapy should be selected.

The cefoxitin disc should be used for testing cefoxitin susceptibility.

Cefoxitin has been shown by *in vitro* tests to have activity against certain strains of *Enterobacteriaceae* found resistant when tested with the cephalosporin class disc. For this reason, the cefoxitin disc should not be used for testing susceptibility to cephalosporins, and cephalosporin discs should not be used for testing susceptibility to cefoxitin.

Dilution methods, preferably the agar plate dilution procedure, are most accurate for sus-

*Bauer, A. W.; Kirby, W. M. M.; Sherris, J. C.; Turck, M.: Antibiotic susceptibility testing by a standardized single disc method, Amer. J. Clin. Path. *45:* 493-496, Apr. 1966. Standardized disc susceptibility test, Federal Register *37:* 20527-20529, 1972. National Committee for Clinical Laboratory Standards: Approved Standard: ASM-2, Performance Standards for Antimicrobial Disc Susceptibility Tests, July 1975.

MEFOXIN®
(Sterile Cefoxitin Sodium)

ceptibility testing of obligate anaerobes.

A bacterial isolate may be considered susceptible if the MIC value for cefoxitin** is not more than 16 mcg/mL. Organisms are considered resistant if the MIC is greater than 32 mcg/mL.

INDICATIONS AND USAGE

Treatment

MEFOXIN is indicated for the treatment of serious infections caused by susceptible strains of the designated microorganisms in the diseases listed below.

(1) **Lower respiratory tract infections,** including pneumonia and lung abscess, caused by *Streptococcus pneumoniae,* other streptococci (excluding enterococci, e.g., *Streptococcus faecalis*), *Staphylococcus aureus* (penicillinase and non-penicillinase producing), *Escherichia coli, Klebsiella* species, *Hemophilus influenzae,* and *Bacteroides* species.

(2) **Genitourinary infections.** Urinary tract infections caused by *Escherichia coli, Klebsiella* species, *Proteus mirabilis,* indole-positive Proteus (which include the organisms now called *Morganella morganii* and *Proteus vulgaris*), and *Providencia* species (including *Providencia rettgeri*). Uncomplicated gonorrhea due to *Neisseria gonorrhoeae* (penicillinase and non-penicillinase producing).

(3) **Intra-abdominal infections,** including peritonitis and intra-abdominal abscess, caused by *Escherichia coli, Klebsiella* species, *Bacteroides* species including the *Bacteroides fragilis* group*, and *Clostridium* species.

(4) **Gynecological infections,** including endometritis, pelvic cellulitis, and pelvic inflammatory disease caused by *Escherichia coli, Neisseria gonorrhoeae* (penicillinase and non-penicillinase producing), *Bacteroides* species including the *Bacteroides fragilis* group*, *Clostridium* species, *Peptococcus* species, *Peptostreptococcus* species, and Group B streptococci.

(5) **Septicemia** caused by *Streptococcus pneumoniae, Staphylococcus aureus* (penicillinase and non-penicillinase producing), *Escherichia coli, Klebsiella* species, and *Bacteroides* species including the *Bacteroides fragilis* group.*

(6) **Bone and joint infections** caused by *Staphylococcus aureus* (penicillinase and non-penicillinase producing).

(7) **Skin and skin structure infections** caused by *Staphylococcus aureus* (penicillinase and non-penicillinase producing), *Staphylococcus epidermidis,* streptococci (excluding enterococci e.g., *Streptococcus faecalis), Escherichia coli, Proteus mirabilis, Klebsiella* species, *Bacteroides* species including the *Bacteroides fragilis* group*, *Clostridium* species, *Peptococcus* species, and *Peptostreptococcus* species.

Appropriate culture and susceptibility studies should be performed to determine the susceptibility of the causative organisms to MEFOXIN. Therapy may be started while awaiting the results of these studies.

In randomized comparative studies, MEFOXIN and cephalothin were comparably safe and effective in the management of infections caused by gram-positive cocci and gram-negative rods susceptible to the cephalosporins. MEFOXIN has a high degree of stability in the presence of bacterial beta-lactamases, both penicillinases and cephalosporinases.

**B. fragilis, B. distasonis, B. ovatus, B. thetaiotaomicron, B. vulgatus.*

**Determined by the ICS agar dilution method (Ericsson and Sherris, Acta Path. Microbiol. Scand. [B] Suppl. No. 217, 1971) or any other method that has been shown to give equivalent results.

Many infections caused by aerobic and anaerobic gram-negative bacteria resistant to some cephalosporins respond to MEFOXIN. Similarly, many infections caused by aerobic and anaerobic bacteria resistant to some penicillin antibiotics (ampicillin, carbenicillin, penicillin G) respond to treatment with MEFOXIN. Many infections caused by mixtures of susceptible aerobic and anaerobic bacteria respond to treatment with MEFOXIN.

Prevention

When compared to placebo in randomized controlled studies in patients undergoing gastrointestinal surgery, vaginal hysterectomy, abdominal hysterectomy and cesarean section, the prophylactic use of MEFOXIN resulted in a significant reduction in the number of postoperative infections.

The prophylactic administration of MEFOXIN may reduce the incidence of certain postoperative infections in patients undergoing surgical procedures (e.g., hysterectomy, gastrointestinal surgery and transurethral prostatectomy) that are classified as contaminated or potentially contaminated.

The perioperative use of MEFOXIN may be effective in surgical patients in whom subsequent infection at the operative site would present a serious risk, e.g., prosthetic arthroplasty.

Effective prophylactic use depends on the time of administration. MEFOXIN usually should be given one-half to one hour before the operation, which is sufficient time to achieve effective levels in the wound during the procedure. Prophylactic administration should usually be stopped within 24 hours since continuing administration of any antibiotic increases the possibility of adverse reactions but, in the majority of surgical procedures, does not reduce the incidence of subsequent infection. However, in patients undergoing prosthetic arthroplasty, it is recommended that MEFOXIN be continued for 72 hours after the surgical procedure.

If there are signs of infection, specimens for culture should be obtained for identification of the causative organism so that appropriate treatment may be instituted.

CONTRAINDICATIONS

MEFOXIN is contraindicated in patients who have shown hypersensitivity to cefoxitin and the cephalosporin group of antibiotics.

WARNINGS

BEFORE THERAPY WITH 'MEFOXIN' IS INSTITUTED, CAREFUL INQUIRY SHOULD BE MADE TO DETERMINE WHETHER THE PATIENT HAS HAD PREVIOUS HYPERSENSITIVITY REACTIONS TO CEFOXITIN, CEPHALOSPORINS, PENICILLINS, OR OTHER DRUGS. THIS PRODUCT SHOULD BE GIVEN WITH CAUTION TO PENICILLIN-SENSITIVE PATIENTS. ANTIBIOTICS SHOULD BE ADMINISTERED WITH CAUTION TO ANY PATIENT WHO HAS DEMONSTRATED SOME FORM OF ALLERGY, PARTICULARLY TO DRUGS. IF AN ALLERGIC REACTION TO 'MEFOXIN' OCCURS, DISCONTINUE THE DRUG. SERIOUS HYPERSENSITIVITY REACTIONS MAY REQUIRE EPINEPHRINE AND OTHER EMERGENCY MEASURES.

Pseudomembranous colitis has been reported with virtually all antibiotics (including

cephalosporins); therefore, it is important to consider its diagnosis in patients who develop diarrhea in association with antibiotic use. This colitis may range from mild to life threatening in severity.

Treatment with broad-spectrum antibiotics alters normal flora of the colon and may permit overgrowth of clostridia. Studies indicate a toxin produced by *clostridium difficile* is one primary cause of antibiotic-associated colitis.

Mild cases of pseudomembranous colitis may respond to drug discontinuance alone. In more severe cases, management may include sigmoidoscopy, appropriate bacteriological studies, fluid, electrolyte and protein supplementation, and the use of a drug such as oral vancomycin as indicated. Isolation of the patient may be advisable. Other causes of colitis should also be considered.

PRECAUTIONS

General

The total daily dose should be reduced when MEFOXIN is administered to patients with transient or persistent reduction of urinary output due to renal insufficiency (see DOSAGE), because high and prolonged serum antibiotic concentrations can occur in such individuals from usual doses.

Antibiotics (including cephalosporins) should be prescribed with caution in individuals with a history of gastrointestinal disease, particularly colitis.

As with other antibiotics, prolonged use of MEFOXIN may result in overgrowth of nonsusceptible organisms. Repeated evaluation of the patient's condition is essential. If superinfection occurs during therapy, appropriate measures should be taken.

Drug Interactions

Increased nephrotoxicity has been reported following concomitant administration of cephalosporins and aminoglycoside antibiotics.

Drug/Laboratory Test Interactions

As with cephalothin, high concentrations of cefoxitin (>100 micrograms/mL) may interfere with measurement of serum and urine creatinine levels by the Jaffé reaction, and produce false increases of modest degree in the levels of creatinine reported. Serum samples from patients treated with cefoxitin should not be analyzed for creatinine if withdrawn within 2 hours of drug administration.

High concentrations of cefoxitin in the urine may interfere with measurement of urinary 17-hydroxy-corticosteroids by the Porter-Silber reaction, and produce false increases of modest degree in the levels reported.

A false-positive reaction for glucose in the urine may occur. This has been observed with CLINITEST* reagent tablets.

Carcinogenesis, Mutagenesis, Impairment of Fertility

Long-term studies in animals have not been performed with cefoxitin to evaluate carcinogenic or mutagenic potential. Studies in rats treated intravenously with 400 mg/kg of cefoxitin (approximately three times the maximum recommended human dose) revealed no effects on fertility or mating ability.

Pregnancy

Pregnancy Category B. Reproduction studies performed in rats and mice at parenteral doses of approximately one to seven and one-half times the maximum recommended human dose did not reveal teratogenic or fetal toxic effects, although a slight decrease in fetal weight was observed.

*Registered trademark of Ames Company, Division of Miles Laboratories, Inc.

There are, however, no adequate and well-controlled studies in pregnant women. Because animal reproduction studies are not always predictive of human response, this drug should be used during pregnancy only if clearly needed.

In the rabbit, cefoxitin was associated with a high incidence of abortion and maternal death. This was not considered to be a teratogenic effect but an expected consequence of the rabbit's unusual sensitivity to antibiotic-induced changes in the population of the microflora of the intestine.

Nursing Mothers

MEFOXIN is excreted in human milk in low concentrations. Caution should be exercised when MEFOXIN is administered to a nursing woman.

Pediatric Use

Safety and efficacy in infants from birth to three months of age have not yet been established. In children three months of age and older, higher doses of MEFOXIN have been associated with an increased incidence of eosinophilia and elevated SGOT.

ADVERSE REACTIONS

MEFOXIN is generally well tolerated. The most common adverse reactions have been local reactions following intravenous or intramuscular injection. Other adverse reactions have been encountered infrequently.

Local Reactions

Thrombophlebitis has occurred with intravenous administration. Pain, induration, and tenderness after intramuscular injections have been reported.

Allergic Reactions

Rash (including exfoliative dermatitis), pruritus, eosinophilia, fever, dyspnea, and other allergic reactions including anaphylaxis and angioedema have been noted.

Cardiovascular

Hypotension

Gastrointestinal

Diarrhea, including documented pseudomembranous colitis which can appear during or after antibiotic treatment. Nausea and vomiting have been reported rarely.

Blood

Eosinophilia, leukopenia including granulocytopenia, neutropenia, anemia, including hemolytic anemia, thrombocytopenia, and bone marrow depression. A positive direct Coombs test may develop in some individuals, especially those with azotemia.

Liver Function

Transient elevations in SGOT, SGPT, serum LDH, and serum alkaline phosphatase; and jaundice have been reported.

Renal Function

Elevations in serum creatinine and/or blood urea nitrogen levels have been observed. As with the cephalosporins, acute renal failure has been reported rarely. The role of MEFOXIN in changes in renal function tests is difficult to assess, since factors predisposing to prerenal azotemia or to impaired renal function usually have been present.

OVERDOSAGE

The acute intravenous LD_{50} in the adult female mouse and rabbit was about 8.0 g/kg and greater than 1.0 g/kg respectively. The acute intraperitoneal LD_{50} in the adult rat was greater than 10.0 g/kg.

DOSAGE

TREATMENT

Adults

The usual adult dosage range is 1 gram to 2

grams every six to eight hours. Dosage and route of administration should be determined by susceptibility of the causative organisms, severity of infection, and the condition of the patient (see Table 1 for dosage guidelines).

MEFOXIN may be used in patients with reduced renal function with the following dosage adjustments:

In adults with renal insufficiency, an initial loading dose of 1 gram to 2 grams may be given. After a loading dose, the recommendations for *maintenance dosage* (Table 2) may be used as a guide.

When only the serum creatinine level is available, the following formula (based on sex, weight, and age of the patient) may be used to convert this value into creatinine clearance. The serum creatinine should represent a steady state of renal function.

$$\text{Males: } \frac{\text{Weight (kg)} \times (140 - \text{age})}{72 \times \text{serum creatinine (mg/100 mL)}}$$

Females: 0.85 x above value

In patients undergoing hemodialysis, the loading dose of 1 to 2 grams should be given after each hemodialysis, and the maintenance dose should be given as indicated in Table 2.

Antibiotic therapy for group A beta-hemolytic streptococcal infections should be maintained for at least 10 days to guard against the risk of rheumatic fever or glomerulonephritis. In staphylococcal and other infections involving a collection of pus, surgical drainage should be carried out where indicated.

The recommended dosage of MEFOXIN **for uncomplicated gonorrhea** is 2 grams intramuscularly, with 1 gram of BENEMID* (Probenecid) given by mouth at the same time or up to 1/2 hour before MEFOXIN.

Infants and Children

The recommended dosage in children three months of age and older is 80 to 160 mg/kg of body weight per day divided into four to six equal doses. The higher dosages should be used for more severe or serious infections. The total daily dosage should not exceed 12 grams.

At this time no recommendation is made for children from birth to three months of age (see PRECAUTIONS).

In children with renal insufficiency the dosage and frequency of dosage should be modified consistent with the recommendations for adults (see Table 2).

PREVENTION

General

For prophylactic use in surgery, the following doses are recommended:

Adults:

(1) 2 grams administered intravenously or intramuscularly just prior to surgery (approximately one-half to one hour before the initial incision).

(2) 2 grams every 6 hours after the first dose for no more than 24 hours (continued for 72 hours after prosthetic arthroplasty).

Children (3 months and older):

30 to 40 mg/kg doses may be given at the times designated above.

Obstetric-Gynecologic

For prophylactic use in vaginal hysterectomy, a single 2.0 gram dose administered intramuscularly one-half to one hour prior to surgery is recommended.

For patients undergoing cesarean section, a single 2.0 gram dose should be administered intravenously as soon as the umbilical cord is clamped. A 3-dose regimen may be more effective than a single dose regimen in preventing postoperative infection (esp. endometritis) following cesarean section. Such a regimen would consist of 2.0 grams given intravenously as soon as the umbilical cord is clamped, followed by 2.0 grams 4 and 8 hours after the initial dose.

Transurethral prostatectomy patients:

One gram administered just prior to surgery; 1 gram every 8 hours for up to five days.

Table 1 — Guidelines for Dosage of MEFOXIN

Type of Infection	Daily Dosage	Frequency and Route
Uncomplicated forms+ of infections such as pneumonia, urinary tract infection, cutaneous infection	3 - 4 grams	1 gram every 6 - 8 hours IV or IM
Moderately severe or severe infections	6 - 8 grams	1 gram every 4 hours *or* 2 grams every 6 - 8 hours IV
Infections commonly needing antibiotics in higher dosage (e.g., gas gangrene)	12 grams	2 grams every 4 hours *or* 3 grams every 6 hours IV

+Including patients in whom bacteremia is absent or unlikely.

Table 2 — Maintenance Dosage of MEFOXIN in Adults with Reduced Renal Function

Renal Function	Creatinine Clearance (mL/min)	Dose (grams)	Frequency
Mild impairment	50 - 30	1 - 2	every 8 - 12 hours
Moderate impairment	29 - 10	1 - 2	every 12 - 24 hours
Severe impairment	9 - 5	0.5 - 1	every 12 - 24 hours
Essentially no function	< 5	0.5 - 1	every 24 - 48 hours

Table 3 — Preparation of Solution

Strength	Amount of Diluent to be Added (mL)++	Approximate Withdrawable Volume (mL)	Approximate Average Concentration (mg/mL)
1 gram Vial	2 (Intramuscular)	2.5	400
2 gram Vial	4 (Intramuscular)	5	400
1 gram Vial	10 (IV)	10.5	95
2 gram Vial	10 or 20 (IV)	11.1 or 21.0	180 or 95
1 gram Infusion Bottle	50 or 100 (IV)	50 or 100	20 or 10
2 gram Infusion Bottle	50 or 100 (IV)	50 or 100	40 or 20
10 gram Bulk	43 or 93 (IV)	49 or 98.5	200 or 100

++Shake to dissolve and let stand until clear.

*Registered trademark of MERCK & CO., INC.

PREPARATION OF SOLUTION

Table 3 is provided for convenience in constituting MEFOXIN for both intravenous and intramuscular administration.

For intravenous use, 1 gram should be constituted with at least 10 mL of Sterile Water for Injection, and 2 grams, with 10 or 20 mL. The 10 gram bulk package should be constituted with 43 or 93 mL of Sterile Water for Injection or any of the solutions listed under the *Intravenous* portion of the COMPATIBILITY AND STABILITY section. CAUTION: THE 10 GRAM BULK STOCK SOLUTION IS NOT FOR DIRECT INFUSION. One or 2 grams of MEFOXIN for infusion may be constituted with 50 or 100 mL of 0.9 percent Sodium Chloride Injection, 5 percent or 10 percent Dextrose Injection, or any of the solutions listed under the *Intravenous* portion of the COMPATIBILITY AND STABILITY section.

Benzyl alcohol as a preservative has been associated with toxicity in neonates. While toxicity has not been demonstrated in infants greater than three months of age, in whom use of MEFOXIN may be indicated, small infants in this age range may also be at risk for benzyl alcohol toxicity. Therefore, diluent containing benzyl alcohol should not be used when MEFOXIN is constituted for administration to infants.

For ADD-Vantage® vials,* see separate INSTRUCTIONS FOR USE OF MEFOXIN IN ADD-Vantage® VIALS. MEFOXIN in ADD-Vantage® vials should be constituted with ADD-Vantage® diluent containers containing 50 mL or 100 mL of either 0.9 percent Sodium Chloride Injection or 5 percent Dextrose Injection. MEFOXIN in ADD-Vantage® vials is for IV use only.

For intramuscular use, each gram of MEFOXIN may be constituted with 2 mL of Sterile Water for Injection, *or—*

For intramuscular use ONLY: each gram of MEFOXIN may be constituted with 2 mL of 0.5 percent lidocaine hydrochloride solution† (without epinephrine) to minimize the discomfort of intramuscular injection.

ADMINISTRATION

MEFOXIN may be administered intravenously or intramuscularly after constitution.

Parenteral drug products should be inspected visually for particulate matter and discoloration prior to administration whenever solution and container permit.

Intravenous Administration

The intravenous route is preferable for patients with bacteremia, bacterial septicemia, or other severe or life-threatening infections, or for patients who may be poor risks because of lowered resistance resulting from such debilitating conditions as malnutrition, trauma, surgery, diabetes, heart failure, or malignancy, particularly if shock is present or impending.

For intermittent intravenous administration, a solution containing 1 gram or 2 grams in 10 mL of Sterile Water for Injection can be injected over a period of three to five minutes. Using an infusion system, it may also be given over a longer period of time through the tubing system by which the patient may be receiving other intravenous solutions. However, during infusion of the solution containing MEFOXIN, it is advisable to temporarily discontinue administration of any other solutions at the same site.

*Registered trademark of Abbott Laboratories, Inc.
†See package circular of manufacturer for detailed information concerning contraindications, warnings, precautions, and adverse reactions.

MEFOXIN®
(Sterile Cefoxitin Sodium)

For the administration of higher doses by continuous intravenous infusion, a solution of MEFOXIN may be added to an intravenous bottle containing 5 percent Dextrose Injection, 0.9 percent Sodium Chloride Injection, 5 percent Dextrose and 0.9 percent Sodium Chloride Injection, or 5 percent Dextrose Injection with 0.02 percent sodium bicarbonate solution. BUTTERFLY* or scalp vein-type needles are preferred for this type of infusion.

Solutions of MEFOXIN, like those of most beta-lactam antibiotics, should not be added to aminoglycoside solutions (e.g., gentamicin sulfate, tobramycin sulfate, amikacin sulfate) because of potential interaction. However, MEFOXIN and aminoglycosides may be administered separately to the same patient.

Intramuscular Administration

As with all intramuscular preparations, MEFOXIN should be injected well within the body of a relatively large muscle such as the upper outer quadrant of the buttock (i.e., gluteus maximus); aspiration is necessary to avoid inadvertent injection into a blood vessel.

COMPATIBILITY AND STABILITY

Intravenous

MEFOXIN, as supplied in vials or the bulk package and constituted to 1 gram/10 mL with Sterile Water for Injection, Bacteriostatic Water for Injection, (see PREPARATION OF SOLUTION), 0.9 percent Sodium Chloride Injection, or 5 percent Dextrose Injection, maintains satisfactory potency for 24 hours at room temperature, for one week under refrigeration (below 5°C), and for at least 30 weeks in the frozen state.

These primary solutions may be further diluted in 50 to 1000 mL of the following solutions and maintain potency for 24 hours at room temperature and at least 48 hours under refrigeration:

Sterile Water for Injection‡
0.9 percent Sodium Chloride Injection
5 percent or 10 percent Dextrose Injection‡
5 percent Dextrose and 0.9 percent Sodium Chloride Injection
5 percent Dextrose Injection with 0.02 percent Sodium Bicarbonate solution
5 percent Dextrose Injection with 0.2 percent or 0.45 percent saline solution
Ringer's Injection
Lactated Ringer's Injection‡
5 percent Dextrose in Lactated Ringer's Injection‡
5 percent or 10 percent invert sugar in water
10 percent invert sugar in saline solution
5 percent Sodium Bicarbonate Injection
Neut (sodium bicarbonate)*‡
M/6 sodium lactate solution
NORMOSOL-M in D5-W*‡
IONOSOL B w/Dextrose 5 percent*‡
POLYONIC M 56 in 5 percent Dextrose**
Mannitol 5% and 2.5%
Mannitol 10%‡
ISOLYTE*** E
ISOLYTE*** E with 5% Dextrose

MEFOXIN, as supplied in infusion bottles and constituted with 50 to 100 mL of 0.9 percent Sodium Chloride Injection, or 5 percent or 10 percent Dextrose Injection, maintains satisfac-

*Registered trademark of Abbott Laboratories, Inc.
‡In these solutions, MEFOXIN has been found to be stable for a period of one week under refrigeration.
**Registered trademark of Cutter Laboratories, Inc.
***Registered trademark of American Hospital Supply Corporation.

tory potency for 24 hours at room temperature or for 1 week under refrigeration (below 5°C).

MEFOXIN is supplied in single dose ADD-Vantage® vials and should be prepared as directed in the accompanying INSTRUCTIONS FOR USE OF MEFOXIN IN ADD-Vantage® VIALS using ADD-Vantage® diluent containers containing 50 mL or 100 mL of either 0.9 percent Sodium Chloride Injection or 5 percent Dextrose Injection. When prepared with either of these diluents, MEFOXIN maintains satisfactory potency for 24 hours at room temperature.

Limited studies with solutions of MEFOXIN in 0.9 percent Sodium Chloride Injection, Lactated Ringer's Injection, and 5 percent Dextrose Injection in VIAFLEX† intravenous bags show stability for 24 hours at room temperature, 48 hours under refrigeration or 26 weeks in the frozen state and 24 hours at room temperature thereafter. Also, solutions of MEFOXIN in 0.9 percent Sodium Chloride Injection show similar stability in plastic tubing, drip chambers, and volume control devices of common intravenous infusion sets.

After constitution with Sterile Water for Injection and subsequent storage in disposable plastic syringes, MEFOXIN is stable for 24 hours at room temperature and 48 hours under refrigeration.

After the periods mentioned above, any unused solutions or frozen material should be discarded. Do not refreeze.

Intramuscular

MEFOXIN, as constituted with Sterile Water for Injection, Bacteriostatic Water for Injection, or 0.5 percent or 1 percent lidocaine hydrochloride solution (without epinephrine), maintains satisfactory potency for 24 hours at room temperature, for one week under refrigeration (below 5°C), and for at least 30 weeks in the frozen state.

After the periods mentioned above, any unused solutions or frozen material should be discarded. Do not refreeze.

MEFOXIN has also been found compatible when admixed in intravenous infusions with the following:

Heparin 0.1 units/mL at room temperature — 8 hours

Heparin 100 units/mL at room temperature — 24 hours

M.V.I.†† concentrate at room temperature 24 hours; under refrigeration 48 hours

BEROCCA††† C-500 at room temperature 24 hours; under refrigeration 48 hours

MEFOXIN®
(Sterile Cefoxitin Sodium)

Insulin in Normal Saline at room temperature 24 hours; under refrigeration 48 hours

Insulin in 10% invert sugar at room temperature 24 hours; under refrigeration 48 hours

HOW SUPPLIED

Sterile MEFOXIN is a dry white to off-white powder supplied in vials and infusion bottles containing cefoxitin sodium as follows:

No. 3356 — 1 gram cefoxitin equivalent
NDC 0006-3356-45 in trays of 25 vials
(6505-01-119-6005, 1 g 25's).

No. 3368 — 1 gram cefoxitin equivalent
NDC 0006-3368-71 in trays of 10 infusion bottles
(6505-01-195-0649, 1 g infusion bottle 10's).

No. 3357 — 2 gram cefoxitin equivalent
NDC 0006-3357-53 in trays of 25 vials
(6505-01-104-6393, 2 g 25's).

No. 3369 — 2 gram cefoxitin equivalent
NDC 0006-3369-73 in trays of 10 infusion bottles
(6505-01-185-2624, 2 g infusion bottle 10's).

No. 3388 — 10 gram cefoxitin equivalent
NDC 0006-3388-67 in trays of 6 bulk bottles
(6505-01-263-0730, 10 g 6's).

No. 3548 — 1 gram cefoxitin equivalent
NDC 0006-3548-45 in trays of 25 ADD-Vantage® vials
(6505-01-262-9509, 1 g ADD-Vantage® 25's).

No. 3549 — 2 gram cefoxitin equivalent
NDC 0006-3549-53 in trays of 25 ADD-Vantage® vials
(6505-01-263-4531, 2 g ADD-Vantage® 25's).

Special storage instructions

MEFOXIN in the dry state should be stored below 30°C. Avoid exposure to temperatures above 50°C. The dry material as well as solutions tend to darken, depending on storage conditions; product potency, however, is not adversely affected.

MERCK SHARP & DOHME, Division of Merck & Co., INC.
West Point, Pa. 19486

†Registered trademark of Baxter International, Inc.
††Registered trademark of USV Pharmaceutical Corp.
†††Registered trademark of Roche Laboratories.

A.H.F.S. Category: 8:12.07

Issued January 1992 DC7057130